Natural Thyroid Care
The Complete Guide to Overcoming Thyroid Problems Physically, Neurologically, and Metabolically

NATURAL THYROID CARE
THE COMPLETE GUIDE TO OVERCOMING THYROID PROBLEMS PHYSICALLY, NEUROLOGICALLY, AND METABOLICALLY

By
Dr. Jeff Smith, D.C.

Disclaimer of Warranties

This book on *Natural Thyroid Care* is purely for informational purposes only. Information in this book does not constitute a contract or agreement of any kind. This book does not affirm that information contained herein is error free, and consequently, will not assume liability for any action taken because of using this information.

We have made every effort to make this book as complete and accurate as possible. However, there may be errors both typographical and in the subject matter. Therefore, the content provided in this book should be used only as a general guide and not as the definitive source of the content covered.

Further, the author and the publisher shall have neither liability nor responsibility to any individual or entity with respect to any damage or loss caused or alleged to be caused directly or indirectly by the information provided in this book.

Foreword

I, Dr. Jeff Smith, have been managing Smith Family Chiropractic & Acupuncture, Inc. in Northwest Arkansas for more than fifteen years. We are experts in varied Chiropractic Techniques like Gonstead, Palmer, BEST, Diversified, Merrick, and similar others. Apart from local clientele, we also cater to patients across Missouri, Oklahoma, Kansas, and Texas.

In addition to typical chiropractic care, massage therapy, and acupuncture, we offer physical therapeutic modalities like muscle stimulation, ultrasound, laser treatment, inferential therapy, intersegmental traction, and TENS. We treat complex medical conditions like severe migraines, fibromyalgia, chronic pain, bulging discs, spinal stenosis, herniated discs, restless leg syndrome, ADHD, vertigo, and radiating or numb pain traveling down arms and legs through brain-based therapies.

About Myself

As a young three-year old boy in California, I had to always carry my inhaler with me and take intermittent allergy shots. My dad's job took us to Oklahoma and thereafter Arkansas. At the age of thirteen, I underwent three years of chiropractic treatment for my allergies under Dr. Harold Pippin at Arkansas. I was completely cured of my allergies. This influenced me a lot.

After completing Bachelor's of Science in Human Biology and Nutrition from the University of Arkansas, I completed my Doctorate in Chiropractic Medicine and Certification in Acupuncture from Cleveland Chiropractic College. I had learned various adjustment techniques of chiropractic medicine from Dr. Harold Pippin while undergoing treatment. This helped me a lot and I could complete my eight-year course within six years. In between, I married and while I attended school, my wife worked at a local chiropractor's office to learn different facets of this business.

I graduated in 1996. In 1998, we started our own chiropractor practice. We were slowly establishing our business when we suffered a serious setback in 2003. A fire devastated almost our entire office. However, x-ray equipment and patients' files were not damaged. Although within a week I started working from my garage, we planned to reestablish our business on our family property. Since then our 'Smith Family Chiropractic & Acupuncture' clinic has been functioning from the same premises.

We have two sons and I expect them to carry forward our chiropractic practice.

Dr. Jeff Smith, D.C.

TABLE OF CONTENTS

Part-I: Introduction

1. Thyroid Diseases - An Overview

Thyroid diseases occur commonly. They affect millions of people and occur with a greater incidence among women. Thyroid diseases affect normal functioning of thyroid gland.

Thyroid is a small butterfly-shaped endocrine gland located in the front of your neck just above your collarbone. The gland is shaped like a butterfly as it encloses your windpipe with its two lobes and is attached through isthmus. The main function of thyroid gland is to produce thyroid hormones. These hormones primarily regulate metabolism of your body. They are also responsible for growth and other important body functions. Thyroid gland uses iodine as available from your diet to produce the hormones. Excess or low levels of the hormones disrupt body functions. Your mental stability and functions could also be disrupted due to changes in thyroid hormone levels.

Thyroxin (T4) and triiodothyronine (T3) are the two most important thyroid hormones produced by thyroid gland. Certain specific cells in thyroid gland produce another hormone, Calcitonin. T3 has greater biological power although constituting only 0.1% of thyroid hormones. T3 affects metabolism functions of all the cells in your body. T4 constitutes 99.9% of thyroid hormones. However, major part of T4 once released from thyroid gland is converted into T3. Calcitonin is not responsible for body metabolism. This hormone regulates calcium levels in your blood.

Functioning of thyroid gland is regulated by pituitary gland located in the brain. Pituitary gland is primarily responsible for regulating the rate of thyroid hormone production and circulation in your body. Pituitary gland is in turn regulated by hypothalamus gland. These three glands are together responsible for production and regulation of thyroid hormones.

Hypothalamus gland releases a hormone, thyrotropin releasing hormone or TRH. This stimulates pituitary gland to release thyroid stimulating hormone or TSH. Next, TSH stimulates thyroid gland to release thyroid hormones. Malfunctioning of any of these glands causes thyroid diseases like hypothyroidism and hyperthyroidism. Hypothyroidism is due to a deficiency of thyroid hormones while hyperthyroidism is due to excess production of thyroid hormones. Hypothyroidism could also occur due to inflammation of thyroid gland, certain medications, or autoimmune diseases. Similarly, hyperthyroidism could be due to Graves' disease, goiter diseases, high iodine levels, or specific medications.

Thyroid diseases do exhibit specific signs and symptoms. However, signs and symptoms vary widely. Severity of hormone deficiency dictates occurrence of specific symptoms. Common symptoms of hypothyroidism include exhaustion with very low energy levels, dry skin, constipation, weight gain, pain in muscles and joints, prolonged or excessive menstrual bleeding, and extreme sensitiveness to cold. Common symptoms of hyperthyroidism include unexplained weight loss, fast heartbeats, extremely sensitive to heat, confusion, delirium, nervousness, irregular menstrual periods or low menstrual bleeding, body tremors, excessive sweating, and increased bowel movements. Hyperthyroidism symptoms are almost absent in mild cases. Often symptoms surface only when the condition worsens. Sometimes, hyperthyroidism could lead to thyroid storm, a fatal condition. Certain thyroid diseases like cysts, enlargement, and cancer occur due to structural problems of thyroid gland. Sometimes thyroid gland enlarges excessively and compresses trachea or esophagus. Such enlargement may affect functioning of lymph nodes.

Blood tests can easily diagnose thyroid diseases. Blood tests detect TSH, T3, and T4 levels. If the test indicates abnormal hormone levels, I would suggest checking of antibody levels in your blood. Specific antibodies include Anti TPO antibodies, Antithyroglobulin antibodies, and TSH receptor stimulating antibodies. If cancer is suspected, I would suggest checking of thyroglobulin levels. If thyroid disease is due to structural problems of gland, I would suggest imaging tests. These include ultrasound of thyroid gland and radioiodine scanning. A thyroid biopsy is done if cancer is suspected.

Thyroid diseases can be easily treated. Common treatment options include medications, radioactive therapy, and surgery. Medications for hypothyroidism include synthetic thyroid hormone to make up for the deficiency. Hyperthyroidism medications lower production of thyroid hormone and treat symptoms like rapid heartbeat. Thyroid hormone replacement, anti-inflammatory medications, and specific steroids can shrink gland size. Radioactive ablation is an option if hyperthyroidism is not responding to medications. Surgery is normally recommended if thyroid gland compresses airway, is cancerous, or to remove overactive nodule. If entire thyroid gland is removed, synthetic thyroid replacement is required. Long-term medications and other treatment options can absolve most thyroid diseases.

===\\\===\\\===\\\===\\\===\\\===\\\===

Part-II: Understanding Thyroid Problems

2. Thyroid Gland - How Does It Work?

Your thyroid gland is a very small gland weighing around twenty to sixty grams. Thyroid gland is surrounded by two fibrous capsules. The outer capsule connects to important nerves and voice box. Inner and outer capsules are connected by loose connective tissue. This allows free movement of thyroid gland and easy change of position.

Thyroid gland consists of two halves called lobes. Each lobe lies along your windpipe. A thin band of thyroid tissue, isthmus, joins both lobes. These lobes contain numerous small vesicles. These are follicles. They store thyroid hormones in the form of small droplets.

The primary function of thyroid gland is to take iodine from your food and convert it into thyroid hormones T3 and T4. Thyroid cells are the only cells in your body that can absorb iodine.

Pituitary gland situated in the brain controls functioning of thyroid gland. When thyroid hormone levels are very low, pituitary gland produces TSH (Thyroid Stimulating Hormone). This stimulates thyroid gland to secrete T3 and T4 thereby raising their levels in blood. When thyroid hormone levels are very high, pituitary gland decreases TSH production thereby restricting thyroid gland functioning. This leads to reduction of T3 and T4 levels in blood.

However, pituitary gland functioning is controlled by hypothalamus in brain. Hypothalamus produces TSH Releasing Hormone or TRH. This instructs pituitary gland as to when to stimulate or restrict the thyroid gland.

===\\\===\\\===\\\===\\\===\\\===\\\===

3. What is a Thyroid Disease?

A thyroid disease is a medical condition resulting from impaired functioning of thyroid gland. Disruption in normal functioning of thyroid gland causes either excess production of thyroid hormones or less production of thyroid hormones. Such disruption occurs due to dysfunction of thyroid gland, pituitary gland, or hypothalamus gland.

Thyroid Diseases

Thyroid diseases include hypothyroidism, hyperthyroidism, anatomical problems, tumors, and other deficiencies. Hypothyroidism affects adults with greater incidence in women and the elderly. Autoimmune thyroid diseases like Graves disease are common in women, although there is no logical reasoning behind such occurrence. They mostly affect teens, young, and middle-aged women.

Hypothyroidism includes Silent thyroiditis, Hashimoto's thyroiditis, acute thyroiditis, Ord's thyroiditis, postoperative hypothyroidism, Thyroid hormone resistance, postpartum thyroiditis, Euthyroid sick syndrome, and Iatrogenic hypothyroidism. Hyperthyroidism includes Graves' disease, Thyroid storm, Plummer's disease, toxic thyroid nodule, and Hashitoxicosis.

Thyroid diseases occurring due to anatomical problems include Goiter like Diffuse goiter, Endemic goiter, and Multinodular goiter, Thyroglossal duct cyst and Lingual thyroid. Thyroid tumors include Thyroid cancer like follicular, papillary, anaplastic, and medullary and Thyroid adenoma. Metastasis and Lymphomas occur in very rare cases.

Cretinism occurs mainly due to severe thyroid deficiency. Specific medications like lithium salts, amiodarone, some types of interferon and IL-2 cause thyroid diseases.

Why does Thyroid disease occur?

When thyroid is overactive, it releases huge amounts of thyroid hormone into bloodstream leading to hyperthyroidism. Your body uses energy much faster than it should and as a result, metabolism rate shoots up.

When thyroid is underactive, it produces and releases very little thyroid hormone into bloodstream leading to hypothyroidism. Your body uses energy slowly and as a result, metabolism rate slows down alarmingly.

Either hyperthyroidism or hypothyroidism could cause thyroid gland to enlarge. If it enlarges excessively, you can feel the lump under your skin in front of your neck. If lump is explicitly seen, it is goiter. Insufficient iodine levels in your diet often enlarge your thyroid gland.

Most thyroid cancers can be treated or controlled with treatment. Sometimes treatment of hyperthyroidism leads to hypothyroidism and you may require thyroid hormone replacement tablets.

===\\\===\\\===\\\===\\\===\\\===\\\===

4. What is Hypothyroidism?

What Is Hypothyroidism?

Hypothyroidism is a specific medical condition resulting from underproduction of thyroid hormone by your thyroid gland. Thyroid hormone levels should be maintained in your body as low levels disrupt metabolic rates in cells. This restricts normal functioning of your body.

Hypothyroidism is derived from Greek words. The prefix hypo means 'under' and thyroidism is derived from Greek words 'thyreos' and 'eidos'. 'Thyreos' means 'shield' and 'eidos' means 'shape or form'.

Who is affected?

Hypothyroidism normally affects women over the age of sixty. Sometimes men also develop this condition. Advanced hypothyroidism occurs if your hypothyroidism remains undiagnosed for a very long period. This is Myxedema. This commonly occurs in adults. Women have a higher incidence to develop this condition. It is a very rare medical condition and can turn fatal. Although hypothyroidism predominantly affects adults only, sometimes children are also affected. Congenital hypothyroidism occurs at birth.

What causes Hypothyroidism?

Causes of Hypothyroidism include:

1. Autoimmune inflammation of thyroid gland or thyroiditis

2. Severe iodine deficiency responsible for decreased production of thyroid hormones

3. Hyperthyroidism treatments like surgery or radiation

4. **Lithium**: Such mood stabilizers are used to treat bipolar disorders. These could cause hypothyroidism. Similar drugs include interleukin-2, interferon alpha, and thalidomide.

5. Pituitary gland disorder

6. **De Quervain's thyroiditis**: A bad flu proves deadly and destroys either a part or whole of your thyroid gland leading to hypothyroidism.

7. **Stress**: Stress may not be a direct cause for hypothyroidism. However, stress is often the cause behind high fluctuations in blood sugar levels and immune problems. Stress increases cortisone levels in blood. This leads to poor conversion of T4 into T3 leading to disruption in thyroid hormone levels in blood.

8. **Pregnancy**: Postpartum thyroiditis leads to hypothyroidism. This could occur until nine months after delivery. It occurs as transient hyperthyroidism followed by transient hypothyroidism. Thyroid returns to normalcy after a period of hyperthyroidism. Sometimes it turns into hypothyroidism. This syndrome is seen in only around five to nine percent of pregnant women. In few cases, thyroxin replacement therapy is required to treat permanent hypothyroidism in such women. Hypothyroidism developed during pregnancy can affect fetus. Congenital hypothyroidism occurs at birth. Such hypothyroidism is very rare and could be due to:

- Severe iodine deficiency in mother's diet during pregnancy
- Iodine deficiency continuing in child after birth

- Absent or defective thyroid gland due to any reason
- Thyroid aplasia or defective hormone metabolism

Thyroid hormone insensitivity is a type of hypothyroidism. However, thyroid hormone levels in such cases are either normal or even at high levels.

What are the risk factors for hypothyroidism?

Common risk factors for hypothyroidism include:

□ Females over fifty years of age
□ Being over sixty years of age
□ Radiation exposure due to any medical treatment
□ Treatment through anti-thyroid drugs or with radioactive iodine
□ Having a close relative with autoimmune disease
□ Partial surgical removal of thyroid gland or Thyroidectomy
□ Iodine deficiency or exposure to iodine-131 leads to absorption of such iodine by thyroid gland. These destroy body cells.

What are the symptoms of Hypothyroidism?

Hypothyroidism upsets chemical balances in body. It does not exhibit any specific symptoms in the early stages. Prolonged untreated hypothyroidism can cause serious health problems like joint pain, obesity, infertility, and heart disease.

Common symptoms include

□ Exhaustion with very low energy levels
□ Constipation
□ Dry skin
□ Weight gain

□ Prolonged or excessive menstrual bleeding
□ Extreme sensitiveness to cold

===\\\===\\\===\\\===\\\===\\\===\\\===

5. The Six Patterns of Low Thyroid Function or Hypothyroidism

There are six patterns to hypothyroidism. Thyroid gland is extremely sensitive and can sense even the minutest change in body chemistry. Further, it accommodates these changes effectively. However, if these changes occur frequently and become chronic in nature, your thyroid gland is no longer sensitive. Common conditions include toxicity, fluctuating blood sugar levels, poor digestion, chronic inflammation, hormonal misbalance, nutritional deficiencies, and adrenal dysfunctions.

Six Hypothyroidism Patterns

1. Thyroid Metabolism
Hypothalamus gland stimulates pituitary gland to release TSH. This stimulates thyroid gland to secrete T3 and T4. These hormones are released in blood through Thyroid Binding Globulin. More than ninety percent of thyroid hormones is in T4 form and should be converted into T3 before cells can use it. Around sixty percent of T4 hormones are converted into T3 in the liver. Further twenty percent of T4 is converted to reverse inactive T3 and is excreted away. The remaining T4 is converted into inactive forms of T3 like T3S and T3AC. Gastrointestinal tract bacteria convert these into active T3. Only thereafter, these hormones help metabolism in body cells.

2. Hypothyroidism Secondary to Pituitary Hypo Function
Sometimes pituitary gland does not supply sufficient TSH to stimulate thyroid gland effectively. TSH levels remain low. Blood test cannot detect hypothyroidism. Rather, low TSH levels indicate

hyperthyroidism. This is a case of suppressed pituitary function. High activity of adrenal hormones sometimes causes pituitary gland to stop functioning. This lowers TSH levels considerably. You develop hypothyroidism symptoms although blood test does not detect it. Thyroid medications could improve symptoms, although I would not advise it. Higher levels of thyroid hormones cause pituitary gland to remain dysfunctional. Further, such high levels of thyroid hormones in blood cause your body cells to become thyroid resistant. Prolonged medication can completely disrupt pituitary and thyroid gland coordination and inter-dependant functional ability. Eventually, you remain dependent on prescription medications permanently.

3. Under-Conversion
In this hypothyroidism pattern, although thyroid and pituitary glands are functioning normally, conversion of inactive T4 into active T3 is not normal. Your body cells are unable to use thyroid hormones available in the blood. However, your blood test remains normal as your thyroid gland is functioning normally. The primary cause for such poor conversion of T4 into T3 is high stress levels. Inflammations and chronic infections also play an important role in poor conversion of T4 into T3. Sometimes impaired liver functions could be the cause behind the problem. In such cases, prescription medications for thyroid may not deliver desirable results. Synthroid is a synthetic form of T4 and a common thyroid prescription medication. This provides temporary relief in such cases. However, your body is still unable to convert T4 into T3 as required by body cells. Nonetheless, thyroid hormones in circulation increase leading to a shutdown of pituitary gland and consequent reactions.

4. Excessive Conversion
This pattern of hypothyroidism is just the opposite of the earlier pattern. Your thyroid and pituitary glands function normally. However, conversion of T4 into T3 is in excess of what is required. High testosterone levels in body accelerate the condition. High T3

levels in body turn your body cells to become resistant to T3. Subsequently, T3 is not absorbed. However, normal TSH levels in blood are recorded in blood tests although you exhibit hypothyroidism symptoms. If you develop this pattern of hypothyroidism, you suffer from accumulated problems of insulin resistance. Increased testosterone levels in women cause polycystic ovary syndrome or PCOS. Prescription thyroid medications do not provide any respite, as T3 levels are already high in blood. In such cases, maintaining blood sugar levels is extremely important.

5. Thyroid Binding Globulin Elevation

TBG or Thyroid binding globulin is a protein that helps transport thyroid hormones through blood. In this pattern, pituitary and thyroid glands function normally and conversion of T4 into T3 is normal. However, TBG is in excess and although TBG transport thyroid hormones, they do not reach requisite body cells as they are in huge numbers. Any free thyroid hormone in the system attaches to a TBG. Nonetheless, body cells do not receive these hormones. Increased levels of TBG could be due to hormone creams, oral contraceptives, food habits, or hormone replacement therapy. TSH levels however remain at normal levels.

6. Thyroid Resistance

Excessive stress causes cortisol levels in blood to increase. Such high levels instigate thyroid resistance. Eventually although TSH levels are normal and T3 levels are normal, hypothyroidism remains undetected. Further, prescription medications do not provide any relief.

Factors that Help Thyroid Functions

Anemia: Those of you with Hashimoto's hypothyroidism are normally anemic. As your body does not have required amount of oxygen, normal body functions of growth, regeneration, and repair is lacking.

Hence, it is important to consider anemic conditions while treating hypothyroidism. Again, anemia could be due to various reasons. Sometimes your body does not respond to iron supplements as red blood cells break down. This causes serious health problems and you should seek immediate medical attention.

Nutritional Factors: A healthy diet is of paramount importance to maintain normal thyroid functions. Intake of essential fatty acids as available in flaxseed, fish oil, black current seed oil, and borage oil is necessary. Restrict intake of hydrogenated and transfats as they do not allow your body metabolize essential fatty acids. Intake of essential vitamins like vitamin A, copper, selenium, magnesium, niacin, and zinc helps in easy conversion of T4 into T3. I would not advise intake of thyroid supplements as they disrupt normal functioning, rather they often cause dysfunction of thyroid gland and others.

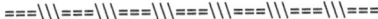

===\\\===\\\===\\\===\\\===\\\===\\\===

6. What is Hyperthyroidism?

What Is Hyperthyroidism?

Hyperthyroidism is when your thyroid gland produces excessive thyroxin or T4. Such high levels of thyroxin in blood push your metabolism rates excessively. This is commonly referred to as overactive thyroid. Graves's disease is the most common form of hyperthyroidism.

What causes Hypothyroidism?

There are many causes responsible for hyperthyroidism. Sometimes your thyroid gland produces excessive thyroxin or a single thyroid nodule secretes huge amounts of thyroxin.

Causes include:

Graves' disease: This autoimmune disease is primarily responsible for hyperthyroidism. Antibodies produced by your immune system stimulate thyroid to produce excess amounts of T-4.

Thyroiditis: Inflammation of thyroid gland causes hyperthyroidism. Different types of thyroiditis include DeQuervain's, Hashimoto's, and others.

Postpartum Thyroiditis: This type of hyperthyroidism is common in women normally within the first year of giving birth to their child. Often such hyperthyroidism does not require any specific treatment as it cures by itself.

Thyroid Hormone Tablets: Excessive consumption of thyroid hormone tablets orally increases thyroxin levels in body leading to hyperthyroidism.

Toxic Adenoma: An adenoma is a part of thyroid gland that has separated due to any reason. Adenomas cause lumps. These lumps produce lots of thyroid hormones leading to hyperthyroidism.

What are the Risk Factors for Hypothyroidism?

Hyperthyroidism is more common in women than in men. If any of your family members has a thyroid problem, you stand a chance of developing hyperthyroidism.

What are the Symptoms of Hypothyroidism?

Hyperthyroidism symptoms do not manifest in the initial stages. Common symptoms include:

- Unexplained weight loss
- Fast heart beats
- Extremely sensitive to heat
- Confusion
- Delirium
- Nervousness
- Irregular menstrual periods or low menstrual bleeding
- Body tremors
- Excessive sweating
- Increased bowel movements

What are the Complications of Hyperthyroidism?

Many medical complications arise due to hyperthyroidism. These include:

Osteoporosis: Bones in your body remain healthy as long as they contain necessary amount of calcium. Excessive thyroxin in blood restricts ability of your body to absorb calcium into your bones. This weakens your bones and they become brittle leading to osteoporosis.

Heart Ailments: Hyperthyroidism causes your heart to beat faster and heart beat rhythms change. Your heart is unable to circulate sufficient blood to all body parts. This leads to congestive heart failure.

Skin and Eye Problems: Graves' disease affects your skin and it turns read and swollen. It also affects your eyes. They turn red, swollen, and sometime bulge out. Vision is affected causing blurring or double vision. Sometimes in severe cases, it causes loss of vision.

Thyrotoxic: In very rare cases, hyperthyroidism leads to sudden crisis. Your pulse rate increases, you develop high fever, and all symptoms manifest extensively. In such instances, I would suggest you to seek immediate medical attention.

Thyroid Storm: Trauma, infection, or injury causes this complication. It is fatal and requires immediate medical help.

How is Hyperthyroidism Diagnosed?

A detailed physical examination and analysis of symptoms can help diagnose hyperthyroidism. Nonetheless, most symptoms do not surface until hyperthyroidism is acute.

Blood tests detect thyroid-stimulating hormone or TSH levels in blood. Low TSH level indicates pituitary gland is restricted from controlling thyroid hormone levels in blood. However, in very rare cases, low TSH levels could be due to pituitary gland failure or any other serious ailment. Hence, it is best to check T3 and T4 levels while diagnosing hyperthyroidism. Sometimes, special diagnostic scan using radioactive iodine uptake is necessary to diagnose hyperthyroidism.

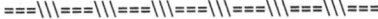

===\\\===\\\===\\\===\\\===\\\===\\\===

7. What are Thyroid Nodules?

What are Thyroid Nodules?

Thyroid nodules are fast evolving as the most common endocrine problem. Any abnormal growth forming a lump in thyroid gland is a thyroid nodule. They develop within a normal thyroid gland. There is no specific cause for development of thyroid nodule. A very meager percentage of thyroid nodules are cancerous.

Thyroid nodule can occur anywhere in the thyroid gland. It is possible to feel nodule within your gland. However, nodules occurring deep within thyroid tissue or lower within the gland cannot be easily felt.

Symptoms

Normally thyroid nodules do not exhibit any specific symptoms. Nonetheless, if cells within nodules function and produce thyroid hormone, it leads to hyperthyroidism. If nodule is very big, it compresses esophagus, causing difficulty in swallowing. Some nodules are painful and pain travels as far as the ear or jaw. In very rare cases, nodules compress larynx leading to choking and hoarseness of voice.

Types of Thyroid Nodules

1. Thyroid nodules are normally non-cancerous in nature. Cancerous nodules could be follicular, papillary, medullary, or anaplastic. Some thyroid nodules contain lymphoma or cancer of immune system.

2. Blood or fluid filled nodule is a thyroid cyst.

3. Thyroid nodules could have single nodule or multiple nodules. Thyroid gland with multiple nodules is a multinodular goiter.

4. Nodule producing unrestricted amounts of thyroid hormone is an autonomous nodule.

Cancerous thyroid nodules are common in people aged more than seventy or less than twenty. Women have more thyroid nodules than men do. Nonetheless, cancerous thyroid nodules occur more in men than in women.

Treatment

Suppressive doses of thyroid therapy can restrict growth of thyroid nodules. Non-cancerous thyroid nodules cause hyperthyroidism. Treatments for such nodules include medications to restrict thyroid production or use of radioactive iodine to destroy gland. However, your age, medical condition, and preferences should be analyzed before choosing any specific treatment for thyroid nodules.

===\\\===\\\===\\\===\\\===\\\===\\\===

8. What is Thyroiditis?

Thyroiditis is a single term applied to different types of individual disorders that cause thyroidal inflammation. Thyroid gland produces hormones that control body metabolism, rate of energy usage, and functioning of your heart. When inflamed, thyroid gland produces and releases excess hormones into the bloodstream. The situation is then similar to hyperthyroid, although a temporary condition.

There are many types of thyroiditis. Each of these types has characteristic features, causes, diagnoses, conditions, durations, risks, and complications. The most common form of thyroiditis is Hashimoto's thyroiditis. This is a major cause of hypothyroidism in the US. Other thyroiditis includes silent thyroiditis, acute thyroiditis same as suppurative thyroiditis, sub acute thyroiditis, postpartum thyroiditis, drug-induced thyroiditis, radiation-induced thyroiditis, and Riedel's thyroiditis.

Symptoms of Hashimoto's thyroiditis are same as that of hypothyroidism. Antibodies cause it. Sub acute thyroiditis same as de Quervain's thyroiditis is caused due to viral infection. Symptoms improve with treatment although sometimes it changes into a case of permanent hypothyroidism. Initial symptoms of silent thyroiditis indicate hyperthyroidism followed by hypothyroidism. Symptoms take around a year and a half to improve. A painful thyroid gland could indicate sub acute thyroiditis. Some women develop postpartum thyroiditis soon after childbirth.

Certain forms of thyroiditis are diagnosed based on tenderness or enlargement of thyroid gland. Thyroiditis can be diagnosed by a biopsy or scan of thyroid gland. Most thyroiditis may result in permanent hypothyroidism.

===\\\===\\\===\\\===\\\===\\\===\\\===

9. What is Thyroid Cancer?

What is Thyroid Cancer?

Thyroid cancer is cancer that starts in the thyroid gland. Although thyroid cancer is not very common in the United States, recent studies indicate an increasing rate of occurrence.

Thyroid cancer starts as a lump or swelling in your neck. Although anyone can develop thyroid cancer, women in the age group of twenty-five to sixty-five are at a greater risk of developing it. If you have a family member with any thyroid disease or if you have had any radiation treatments in neck and head, chances of developing thyroid cancer increase.

There are different types of thyroid cancer. They include:

Papillary
This is the most common type. It starts developing slowly in follicular cells. Early diagnosis ensures complete cure.

Follicular
This is similar to papillary thyroid cancer. However, it is less common than papillary cancer.

Medullary
This thyroid cancer is very rare. It begins in C cells and increases calcitonin levels alarmingly. It grows slowly and can be cured if detected early. Often, such cancer is hereditary.

Anaplastic

This is an extremely rare form of cancer. It starts in follicular cells of thyroid and spreads very fast. It is difficult to control its growth.

Treatment depends on type and severity of thyroid cancer. Options include hormone treatment, surgery, chemotherapy, radioactive iodine, radiation therapy, or a combination of treatments. Normally thyroid cancer can be cured.

===\\\===\\\===\\\===\\\===\\\===\\\===

10. What is a Goiter?

Goiter is a medical condition occurring due to enlargement of thyroid gland (thyromegaly). This causes swelling of larynx (voice box) or neck. The word goiter comes from Latin word 'gutteria'. Presence of goiter does not mean your thyroid gland is not functioning. Goiter only indicates a specific condition that is causing thyroid to grow abnormally.

Lack of adequate iodine in your diet is the primary cause for goiter. More than ninety percent of goiters across the world are due to iodine deficiency. Nonetheless, goiter sometimes occurs due to nodules developing in thyroid gland, cancerous cells in thyroid gland, excess secretion of thyroid hormones or underproduction of thyroid hormones.

Hormone production in thyroid gland is controlled by pituitary gland. This gland releases TSH to prompt thyroid to produce T3 and T4. However, thyroid cannot secrete these hormones without sufficient iodine. If you consume less iodine, your thyroid gland cannot produce hormones despite continuous prompts through chemical messages by pituitary gland. This leads to enlargement of thyroid gland.

Goiters are either endemic or sporadic. Endemic goiters affect a whole community normally across mountainous areas or regions far away from sea. Sporadic affect specific individuals only. Women are more susceptible to goiter.

Most goiters are painless. Some large goiters could pose problems in swallowing or breathing. Small goiters often go unnoticed, as they are too small. Treatment depends on size of goiter, your symptoms, and underlying causes.

===\\\===\\\===\\\===\\\===\\\===\\\===

11. Causes and Evaluation of Hypothyroidism

Insufficient production of thyroid hormones leads to hypothyroidism.

Causes of Hypothyroidism

Causes for hypothyroidism include:

Hyperthyroidism Treatment

Hyperthyroidism occurs due to excessive production of thyroid hormones by thyroid gland. Anti-thyroid medications or radioactive iodine can reduce these high levels of thyroid hormones. However, sometimes such treatments reduce thyroid hormones levels much below normal levels. This leads to hypothyroidism.

Autoimmune Disease

Immune system produces antibodies to fight away infection. When these antibodies instead attack your body tissues, it is autoimmune disease. Hashimoto's thyroiditis is an autoimmune disease. As a result, your thyroid gland is unable to produce sufficient amount of hormones leading to hypothyroidism.

Medications

Certain medications like lithium used to treat mental disorders affect thyroid gland functioning. Often it lowers hormone production leading to hypothyroidism.

Radiation Therapy

Radiation treatments are used to cure cancers of head or neck. These treatments affect functioning of thyroid gland leading to hypothyroidism.

Surgery

Surgical removal of a part or whole of thyroid gland disrupts hormone production in thyroid gland. Hormone production sometimes stops. These conditions lead to hypothyroidism.

Pregnancy

Some women produce antibodies during or after pregnancy. These antibodies affect their own thyroid gland. This leads to hypothyroidism. It also causes other complications like miscarriage, high blood pressure and can affect the growing fetus.

Iodine Deficiency

Trace amounts of iodine are necessary for production of thyroid hormones in body. When your diet lacks iodine content, you develop hypothyroidism as your thyroid gland produces insufficient amounts of thyroid hormones.

Pituitary Disorder

Pituitary gland monitors functioning of thyroid gland. It produces TSH or thyroid stimulating hormone that instructs thyroid gland to produce hormones and maintain normal hormonal levels. Sometimes cancers or tumors in pituitary gland restrict its functioning. As a result, pituitary gland produces insufficient amounts of TSH. Consequently, thyroid gland produces lesser hormones leading to hypothyroidism.

Congenital Disease

Some babies are born without a thyroid gland or with a deformed thyroid gland for unknown reasons. In both cases, thyroid gland is unable to secrete hormones leading to hypothyroidism. However, such babies look normal at birth.

Radiation Exposure

If you live close to nuclear power plants or are exposed to radiation effects, your body absorbs iodine-131 just like regular iodide. Iodine-131 is harmful and destroys cells in thyroid gland. This obstructs normal production of hormones leading to hypothyroidism.

Stress

Stress is a major contributor to thyroid dysfunction. It leads to hypothyroidism as stress reduces conversion of T4 into T3. Hence, there is a shortage of thyroid hormones. Chronic stress accumulates in your body and often leads to subclinical hypothyroidism, a very high rate of hypothyroidism.

Adrenal Insufficiency

Adrenal insufficiency also leads to hypothyroidism, although it does not affect the thyroid gland itself.

Evaluation of Hypothyroidism

Hypothyroidism affects elderly women, rather women over the age of sixty. It also sometimes affects pregnant women within the first year of giving birth. If your parent or grandparent has any autoimmune disease, you are at a greater risk of developing hypothyroidism. If you have been treated with anti-thyroid medications, radioactive iodine, or have undergone radiation therapy in the upper part of your body, you could develop hypothyroidism.

Normally, a simple blood test diagnoses hypothyroidism. In some cases, few more tests that are detailed are necessary. Hypothyroidism is completely treatable. There is no single treatment option that works for all hypothyroidism patients. Nonetheless, if hypothyroidism symptoms are left untreated, it could lead to severe consequences like depression, coma, and heart failure.

===\\\===\\\===\\\===\\\===\\\===\\\===

12. Causes and Evaluation of Hyperthyroidism

Your thyroid gland produces two main hormones. These are thyroxin or T4 and triiodothyronine or T-3. These hormones are essential to maintain normal functioning of body cells. Pituitary gland and hypothalamus in your brain monitor the rate at which these hormones are released into your bloodstream. Pituitary gland releases thyroid-stimulating hormone or TSH depending on amount of thyroid hormones in circulation. Normally, thyroid gland releases correct amount of hormones into bloodstream. Sometimes it produces excessive T-4. This leads to hyperthyroidism.

Causes of Hyperthyroidism

Causes for hyperthyroidism include:

Diffuse Toxic Goiter or Graves disease
This is the most common cause for hyperthyroidism. More than 95% of people with hyperthyroidism are diagnosed with Graves's disease. This is an autoimmune disorder. Normally immune system produces antibodies to protect you against bacteria, viruses, and other infections. In autoimmune disorder, antibodies produced by your body act against your immune system. These antibodies stimulate your thyroid gland to produce large amounts of T4. This leads to hyperthyroidism.

Toxic Adenoma
Nodules form within thyroid gland. Often these nodules are harmless. Sometimes a single nodule suddenly becomes overactive and produces

excessive thyroid hormone. This is termed a hot nodule. This leads to hyperthyroidism. At times, many nodules within thyroid become overactive and produce hormones in excess. This enlarges thyroid leading to multinodular goiter or Plummer's disease. Eventually it causes hyperthyroidism.

Thyroiditis

Thyroiditis is a disease of thyroid gland. Your thyroid gland inflames or enlarges for no apparent reason. Enlargement causes excess thyroid hormones stored in thyroid gland to leak into bloodstream. This causes hyperthyroidism. There are different types of thyroiditis. Most are painless. Sub acute thyroiditis is a rare type of thyroiditis. This causes lot of pain in thyroid gland. Some women develop postpartum thyroiditis within the first year of giving birth. This thyroiditis passes through different phases, first being hyperthyroidism. Eventually, this condition normalizes without medical treatment.

Medications and Drugs

Certain drugs like Amiodarone stimulate thyroid gland to produce more hormones leading to hyperthyroidism. Iodine containing drugs increase body iodine levels to alarming levels leading to hyperthyroidism.

Thyroid Hormone Tablets

Oral consumption of thyroid hormone tablets in excess increases hormone levels in bloodstream leading to hyperthyroidism. In extremely rare occurrences, consumption of ground beef contaminated with thyroid tissue increases hormone levels in bloodstream. This is hamburger hyperthyroidism.

Tumors

Sometimes, tumors develop in ovaries or pituitary gland. These produce thyroid hormones in excess leading to hyperthyroidism.

Evaluation of Hyperthyroidism

Hyperthyroidism requires medical attention. At times symptoms worsen suddenly due to stress or infection. This causes abdominal pain, decreased mental alertness, and fever. This is thyroid crisis or thyrotoxicosis. I recommend immediate hospitalization in such cases. Hyperthyroidism could increase heart rate excessively leading to congestive heart failure. Prolonged hyperthyroidism causes bones to become brittle leading to osteoporosis.

===\\\===\\\===\\\===\\\===\\\===\\\===

13. Causes and Evaluation of Thyroid Nodules

Causes of Thyroid Nodules

Causes of thyroid nodules are various. These include:

Growth of thyroid tissue
Sometimes cells in thyroid gland start growing uncontrollably. These are thyroid nodules or adenomas. Normally, they are non-cancerous. Sometimes these nodules or adenomas start producing hormones without adhering to pituitary gland control. Hormone levels increase leading to hyperthyroidism.

Thyroiditis
Thyroiditis is chronic inflammation of thyroid gland. This leads to inflammation and enlargement of thyroid gland. Gland activity reduces and nodules form within gland.

Genetic Factors
Sometimes certain genes cause nodules to form within thyroid gland.

Radiation Exposure
If you have undergone radiation treatment in head or neck for any other ailment, nodules could develop within your thyroid gland.

Thyroid Cyst
Disintegrating thyroid adenomas may cause cavities filled with fluid and solid particles within thyroid gland. Although such cysts are non-cancerous, sometimes they turn malignant.

Iodine Deficiency

Insufficient iodine in diet causes thyroid gland to enlarge and produce nodules. This is goiter. Multinodular goiter contains many distinct nodules within itself.

Thyroid Cancer

Hard or large nodules are sometimes painful. These nodules could turn malignant leading to thyroid cancer.

Evaluation of Thyroid Nodules

There is no specific cause for growth and development of thyroid nodules. Nonetheless, if you develop such nodules, it may lead to cancer if nodules turn malignant for any reason. If nodules disrupt normal hormone production within thyroid gland, it could lead to hypothyroidism or hyperthyroidism.

===\\\===\\\===\\\===\\\===\\\===\\\===

14. Causes and Evaluation of Thyroiditis

Causes of Thyroiditis

Causes of thyroiditis include:

Malfunction of Immune System

Malfunction of immune system leads to thyroiditis. Antibodies attack thyroid as if thyroid gland is a foreign tissue in your body. This inflames and damages thyroid cells.

Viral or Bacterial Infection

Viral or bacterial infection affects cells in thyroid gland leading to thyroiditis.

Drugs

Certain drugs like amiodarone and interferon damage thyroid cells thereby causing thyroiditis.

When thyroid gland functions normally, hormones are released into bloodstream in a regulated manner. When bacteria, antibodies, or viruses inflame thyroid gland, hormone release is hampered. T4 levels in blood increase excessively and your thyroid gland stops production of T4. Eventually, gland loses its ability to produce T4. This is a case of underactive thyroid. As a result, hypothyroidism and thyroiditis develop.

Evaluation of Thyroiditis

Thyroiditis is due to an attack on your thyroid gland. It is more common in women than in men. Women are three to five times more likely to develop thyroiditis than men are. It occurs primarily in summer and fall. Thyroiditis shows geographical-specific characteristics. Women in the age range of thirty to fifty years have a higher chance of developing thyroiditis.

I physically examine and palpate thyroid gland to diagnose thyroiditis. Blood tests determine thyroid levels and presence of antibodies in blood. This helps diagnose type of thyroiditis. At times, I advise a biopsy to detect what is attacking your thyroid gland.

===\\\===\\\===\\\===\\\===\\\===\\\===

15. Causes and Evaluation of Thyroid Cancer

Causes of Thyroid Cancer

There are no clear clues for occurrence of thyroid cancer. Cells in thyroid gland undergo changes or mutations for no specific reason. These changes prompt cells to grow and multiply very fast. Normally, body cells die by themselves. However, cells undergoing mutation lose their ability to die. Numerous cells start accumulating in thyroid gland. These form into a tumor or cancer. Such abnormal cells affect other tissues in the vicinity. Slowly they spread all over the body. Thyroid cancer can be treated.

In acute cases of thyroid cancer, I advise removal of thyroid. Despite this, it is possible for recurrence of thyroid cancer. Microscopic cancer cells spread beyond the thyroid much before it is removed. These cells recur as thyroid cancer much later, sometimes even after two or three decades.

Evaluation of Thyroid Cancer

It is not possible to pinpoint actual cause of thyroid cancer. If you or your family members have goiter, a noncancerous enlargement of thyroid, you could develop thyroid cancer. If you live close to high radiation places like weapons testing, nuclear power plants, you have greater chance of developing thyroid cancer. If you undergo radiation treatments in head or neck, you might test positive for thyroid cancer. If you have a family history of multiple endocrine neoplasia, familial medullary thyroid cancer, and familial adenomatous polyposis, possibility of developing thyroid cancer is high.

===\\\===\\\===\\\===\\\===\\\===\\\===

16. Causes and Evaluation of Goiter

Causes of Goiter

There is no specific reason for occurrence of a simple goiter. Often small goiters go unnoticed, as they do not form a lump in throat. If you have goiter, it does not mean that your thyroid gland is not working normally. An enlarged thyroid may produce normal amounts of hormones. Sometimes it could produce excess hormones while sometimes it could produce insufficient hormones.

Common factors that cause your thyroid gland to enlarge include:

Hyperthyroidism
Your thyroid gland produces excessive amounts of thyroid hormones. This causes gland to swell and form goiter.

Iodine Deficiency
Insufficient iodine in your diet causes goiter. Although iodine is in abundance along coastal regions, if you live inland, I suggest you should include iodine in your daily diet in the form of table salt and other foods. Restrict consumption of hormone inhibiting foods like broccoli, cabbage, and cauliflower.

Hashimoto's Disease
This is an autoimmune disease. It damages your thyroid gland such that hormone production is severely affected. Low hormone levels prompt pituitary gland to release more TSH to stimulate thyroid gland. This enlarges thyroid, which may cause goiter.

Graves' Disease

This is an autoimmune disease. Antibodies produced by your immune system attack your thyroid gland and it produces excess thyroxin. This causes thyroid to swell and develop goiter.

Pregnancy

Human chorionic gonadotropin or HCG is a hormone produced during pregnancy. This enlarges thyroid gland, although marginally.

Thyroid Nodule

A single nodule forms within thyroid gland for no apparent reason. This enlarges thyroid leading to goiter. Often such nodules are non-cancerous.

Multinodular Goiter

Sometimes numerous nodules develop in both sides of your thyroid. These contain fluid or solid particles. They enlarge gland leading to goiter.

Thyroid Cancer

At time, nodules formed within thyroid gland are cancerous. This enlarges thyroid gland on one side.

Evaluation of Goiter

A simple goiter may disappear by itself. Small goiters do not cause any serious problems. Sometimes goiters become toxic and produce hormones leading to hyperthyroidism. Sometimes goiters enlarge such that they compress your windpipe or esophagus. This leads to difficulties in swallowing or breathing.

===\\\===\\\===\\\===\\\===\\\===\\\===

17. Who are at Risk for Getting a Thyroid Disease?

Risk Factors for Thyroid Disease

Age
Men and women over the age of fifty have a greater risk of developing thyroid disorders.

Gender
Women are at a greater risk of thyroid problems than men are. Women are six to eight times more susceptible to thyroid disorders. Graves' disease affects women in the age group of twenty and sixty. Hence, even young women with Graves' disease could develop thyroid problems.

Family History
If your mother, sister, or any other female relative has thyroid problems, you stand a greater risk of developing it sometime in your life. Similarly, if any of your close relatives has any autoimmune disease like Graves' disease or Hashimoto's disease, you could develop thyroid problems.

Radioactive Iodine Treatment (RAI)
This treatment could progress into hypothyroidism. This is a common treatment option for hyperthyroidism.

Personal History
If you have had any thyroid problems and undergone treatment, there is every chance of reoccurrence. If postpartum thyroiditis resolved

soon after pregnancy, you could develop a thyroid problem sometime later in life too.

Pregnancy

You stand an increased risk of developing thyroiditis or any autoimmune disease that could lead to thyroid disorders during pregnancy or in the first year of childbirth.

Thyroid Surgery

Surgical removal of thyroid causes hypothyroidism as thyroid secretion is either too low or nil.

Smoking

Cigarettes contain a chemical, thiocyanate. This acts as an anti-thyroid agent and affects thyroid gland adversely. Hormone secretion is disrupted. Smoking affects your eyes as it further complicates eye problems caused due to Graves' disease. It also increases severity of side effects of Hashimoto thyroiditis. Although risk is considerably reduced if you quit smoking, yet you stand a greater chance of developing thyroid disorders in comparison to a nonsmoker.

Medications

Certain drugs and medications like Interleukin-4, antiretrovirals, immunosuppressants, Interferon Beta-1b, lithium, and amiodarone increase the risk of thyroid disorders. Treatment options like bone marrow transplant and other treatments to cure cancer of head and neck also cause thyroid problems.

Surgical Antiseptic Exposure

Surgical antiseptic contains iodine. This is commonly used during surgery. If you have an underlying thyroid problem, surgical iodine could cause temporary hyperthyroidism, hypothyroidism, or thyroiditis.

Presence or Absence of Iodine

Iodine deficiency causes thyroid disorders. If you live in mountainous regions or extremely inland and if you do not include sufficient iodine in your diet, you develop goiter and hypothyroidism. If you regularly consume iodine supplements despite being iodine-sufficient, you are at a risk of developing hyperthyroidism due to high concentrations of iodine. Hence, excess or insufficient iodine levels are responsible for thyroid disorders.

Goitrogenic Foods

Goitrogenic foods if eaten raw and in large quantities, may cause goiter and other thyroid problems. Goitrogenic foods include broccoli, radish, turnip, cauliflower, Brussels sprouts, cabbage, kale, and millet. Soy foods as found in concentrated forms in powders or pills also pose risk of developing thyroid problems. Soy foods hamper thyroid hormone absorption.

Stress

Stress of any kind is a risk factor for thyroid problems. Major life events like death, accident, divorce, and similar others cause mental stress and agony. This makes you susceptible to thyroid problems. Further, if you already have any underlying thyroid problems, they manifest under such stressful conditions.

Genetic Factors

Specific genetic factors cause you to be ambidextrous, prematurely gray, or left-handed. These factors could also cause thyroid disorders, although there is no definite and conclusive proof.

===\\\===\\\===\\\===\\\===\\\===\\\===

18. Signs and Symptoms of Hypothyroidism

Symptoms of hypothyroidism in the initial stages are very subtle and often go unnoticed. These symptoms are similar to symptoms of various other ailments. Further, some of you may not have any symptoms at all. Every individual exhibits either one or many symptoms depending on the deficiency level of thyroid hormone and the length of time since the deficiency has set in. Often symptoms develop slowly and gradually over a number of years.

Common symptoms of hypothyroidism include:

- Unexplained weight gain
- Slowed heart rate, fewer than sixty beats per minute, causing fatigue and exhaustion
- Constipation
- Increased sensitivity to cold
- Dry and itchy skin
- Muscle aches, cramps, stiffness, and tenderness leading to muscular weakness
- Irregular menstrual periods and infertility
- Thinning of hair
- Hoarseness of voice
- Puffy face due to water retention
- High blood cholesterol levels
- Pain in joints
- Thin and brittle fingernails
- Decreased sweating

If hypothyroidism symptoms are not treated promptly, condition worsens. Insufficient hormones levels in blood prompt pituitary gland to send more TSH to thyroid gland. Such constant stimulation enlarges thyroid leading to goiter. Your brain functions are impaired and your thought process slows down. Your memory levels drop. You go into depression. Your speech is incoherent and voice is muffled. Stress develops and you are prone to sudden mood swings. Men develop low libido. Sometimes hypothyroidism causes deafness, an enlarged tongue, decreased sense of taste and smell, accumulation of water in lungs or pleurisy, and impaired renal functions.

In very rare instances, hypothyroidism turns fatal. This condition is termed Myxedema. Symptoms of this condition include:

□ Decreased body temperature
□ Low blood pressure
□ Decreased breathing,
□ Unresponsiveness progressing into coma

Symptoms of Hypothyroidism in Infants

Hypothyroidism normally affects middle-aged and elderly women. However, infants can develop this condition. Some infants are born with an inactive thyroid gland or even without a thyroid gland. Hypothyroidism symptoms in infants include:

□ Large, protruding tongue
□ Puffy face
□ Yellowing of skin and eyes as liver is unable to metabolize bilirubin due to low or no thyroid hormones
□ Frequent choking

As hypothyroidism continues, infants do not grow normally as they are unable to feed properly. They sleep for long hours and have weak muscles. If untreated, it could lead to serious physical and mental retardation.

Symptoms of Hypothyroidism in Children and Teens

Symptoms are often the same as those experienced by adults. In addition, children and teenagers exhibit few additional symptoms. These include:

▫ Short stature due to poor physical growth
▫ Poor mental development
▫ Delayed development of permanent teeth
▫ Delayed puberty

Correct and prompt diagnosis of hypothyroidism can correct all symptoms through proper treatments and medications.

===\\\===\\\===\\\===\\\===\\\===\\\===

19. Signs and Symptoms of Hyperthyroidism

When your thyroid gland produces excessive amounts of T3 and T4, it is hyperthyroidism. These hormones are responsible for body metabolic processes. Hence, excess amounts of these hormones increase body metabolic rate. Thyroid hormone is important for every function of body cells. Hence, changes in thyroid hormone levels affect almost all the different body processes. If there is excess thyroid hormone in body, body functions accelerate. Metabolic rate shoots up, nervous functions speed up, and you feel confused, irritated, and shaken.

There are various signs and symptoms of hyperthyroidism. Not everyone with hyperthyroidism will exhibit all symptoms. Often, some do not experience any symptoms at all. Symptoms vary according to your age, how long you have been experiencing such symptoms, your medical conditions, and others.

Common hyperthyroidism symptoms include:

- Increased appetite
- Sudden loss of weight although food intake remains same
- Nervousness, irritability, and anxiety
- Excessive heat intolerance
- Rapid heartbeat as high as hundred per minute
- Trembling of hands and fingers
- Changes in menstrual patterns
- Excessive sweating
- Insomnia
- Thinning of hair

▫ Muscular weakness
▫ Tiredness and fatigue
▫ Enlarged thyroid gland or goiter
▫ Frequent bowel movements
▫ High blood pressure
▫ Breast development in men
▫ Itching sensation all over the body
▫ Clammy skin
▫ Nausea and vomiting
▫ Lower leg swelling
▫ Shortness of breath with exertion
▫ Sudden paralysis
▫ Irregular heartbeat
▫ Breathing problems even while resting
▫ Impaired fertility
▫ Changes in vision with light sensitivity, irritation of eyes, double vision, regular formation of tears in eyes
▫ Staring gaze
▫ Graves's disease leads to hyperthyroidism. People with this disease have huge bulging eyes. Eye muscles swell and push eye forward, almost out of the socket. Surgical treatment can compress eyeballs to a certain extent. Those with Graves's disease experience additional symptoms like:

▫ thick nails that lift off their bed
▫ goiter
▫ clubbing or fingers with wide tips
▫ reddish, lumpy, and thick skin on top of feet or front of chin
▫ fluid buildup in tissues around chin

Hyperthyroidism symptoms left untreated could cause severe complications. It culminates into high fever and dehydration, sudden increase in body temperature to as high as 104 degrees Fahrenheit, vomiting, coma, and eventual death. This is thyroid storm. This requires immediate hospitalization and medical treatment to lower circulation of thyroid hormone levels and restrict further production. Although presently this is a rare occurrence due to intensive therapy, thyroid storm is fatal in nature.

Normally hyperthyroidism symptoms manifest similarly across all. Nonetheless, hyperthyroidism symptoms have a significant effect on the elderly as they already suffer from various age-related ailments. Further, complications from different ailments often develop a confusing scenario with overlapping symptoms. Diagnosis also takes more time as they have to undergo various tests to determine what the actual ailment is. Often medications for high blood pressure like beta-blockers hide most hyperthyroidism symptoms in the elderly. If left untreated, hyperthyroidism assume serious complications, sometimes even leading to osteoporosis.

If you experience any of the symptoms of hyperthyroidism, it is essential to explain everything in full detail to your doctor. You would remain under observation for few days. You also undergo different tests. Only then, it is possible to arrive at the exact medical ailment. Once you start hyperthyroidism treatment, visit your doctor regularly, and follow all medical advice diligently. Only then, it is possible to regulate and stabilize your condition.

===\\\===\\\===\\\===\\\===\\\===\\\===

20. Signs and Symptoms of Thyroid Nodules

Most thyroid nodules are too small. They cannot be felt and have to be seen under a microscope. Often a CT scan, ultrasound, or routine physical examination detects thyroid nodules. Thyroid nodule may be present as a single swelling in gland. This is solitary nodule. Sometimes it is a dominant nodule. Most nodules are benign or non-cancerous.

Thyroid nodules do not normally exhibit any symptoms. If nodules become big, they compress neck tissue. Symptoms develop like:

▫ Enlarged thyroid or goiter
▫ Clearly visible lump in throat
▫ Rapidly growing lump in neck
▫ Pain in the neck
▫ Difficulty in swallowing
▫ Difficulty in breathing
▫ Change in voice quality with voice turning hoarse
▫ Enlargement of lymph nodes and other glands in throat

Sometimes thyroid nodules produce thyroid hormones. This leads to excess hormones or hyperthyroidism. Common symptoms of hormone producing thyroid nodules include:

▫ Increased appetite
▫ Rapid or irregular heartbeat leading to fast pulse
▫ Moist and damp skin
▫ Restlessness
▫ Nervousness

▫ Weight loss

Sometimes thyroid nodules disrupt production of thyroid hormones. This causes hormone levels to fall leading to hypothyroidism. Common symptoms include:

▫ Excessive tiredness or fatigue
▫ Unable to bear cold temperatures
▫ Dry skin
▫ Hair loss
▫ Swelling of face
▫ Weight gain for no apparent reason
▫ Forgetfulness
▫ Constipation
▫ Depression

===\\\===\\\===\\\===\\\===\\\===\\\===

21. Signs and Symptoms of Thyroiditis

Thyroiditis refers to various disorders of thyroid gland. Hence, signs and symptoms vary according to type of thyroiditis.

If thyroid cell damage is slow and chronic, symptoms are same as that of hypothyroidism. These include:

□ Weight gain
□ Fatigue
□ Dry skin
□ Depression
□ Constipation
□ Decreased concentration levels
□ Swelling of legs
□ Body pain

In severe cases, symptoms include:

□ Drop in body temperature
□ Puffiness around the eyes
□ Slowing of heart rate
□ Eventual heart failure

If thyroid cell damage is intense, symptoms are same as that of hyperthyroidism. These include:

□ Weight loss
□ Insomnia
□ Irritability
□ Fast heart rate

▫ Anxiety
▫ Fatigue

If thyroid cell damage is extremely severe, hormones from thyroid gland leak into bloodstream. Hormone levels are then excessively high. This condition is termed thyrotoxicosis. It is not hyperthyroidism as high levels of hormones in blood is not due to excessive secretion of thyroid gland. The high levels are due to damage of thyroid gland and eventual leakage of hormones.

Other symptoms of thyroiditis include:
▫ Pain in the jaw, neck, or ear
▫ Influenza
▫ Upper respiratory infections
▫ Mumps
▫ Enlargement of thyroid gland
▫ Inability to tolerate cold temperatures
▫ Stiffening of joints stiffen
▫ Tremors
▫ Feeling instable and confused
▫ Rapid heartbeat
▫ Feverish
▫ Extreme Tiredness
▫ Nervousness

===\\\===\\\===\\\===\\\===\\\===\\\===

22. Signs and Symptoms of Thyroid Cancer

In the early stages of thyroid cancer, often there are no symptoms at all. Doctors detect a nodule or lump in your neck during a routine physical examination and advice tests. Sometimes symptoms surface as thyroid cancer grows.

Signs and symptoms of thyroid cancer include:

Lump in the Neck
You see a small lump or a protrusion in the neck within thyroid gland.

Voice Change
Sound of your voice changes into a hoarser tone. Voice turns hoarse due to paralysis of vocal folds. You find it difficult to talk in your normal voice.

Swollen Lymph Nodes
Lymph nodes enlarge. It is common to have many small nodules in thyroid gland. Sometimes, a very small percentage of these nodules, turn malignant, grow in size, and start multiplying uncontrollably.

Difficulty in Swallowing or Breathing
Overgrown cells compress esophagus and windpipe. You find it difficult to swallow and to breathe normally.

Persistent Cough and Cold
You develop a nagging sore throat and cold. Despite medications, sore throat does not improve. You continue to cough and experience discomfort in throat. Often, this translates into a constant pain in

throat and neck. Sometimes pain travels to your ears. Nerves in the neck are compressed by the growing cancerous cells.

Sometimes, severe thyroid tumors may affect brain and its associated neurological functions. When thyroid cancer symptoms worsen, weight loss is distinct.

===\\\===\\\===\\\===\\\===\\\===\\\===

23. Signs and Symptoms of Goiter

Signs and Symptoms of Goiter

Goiters do not always exhibit symptoms. Some goiters are present without any symptoms at all. Nonetheless, characteristic symptoms of goiters include:

A clearly visible swelling at base of your neck: This is the primary symptom. Swelling could be as small as a nodule or as large as a lump in throat.

Coughing more often than usual: Lump causes an irritating feeling in throat. You cough often to clear your throat.

Tight feeling in throat: You feel a lump moving up and down your throat. This constricts your throat leading to a feeling of tightness.

Difficulty in swallowing: Swollen thyroid compresses against esophagus. Hence, you are unable to swallow easily.

Difficulty in breathing normally: Swollen thyroid puts pressure on your windpipe. This restricts easy flow of air and you find it difficult to breathe normally.

Hoarseness of voice: Excessive coughing and compression of voice box makes your voice sound hoarse.

Goiter at times occurs due to very low (hypothyroidism) or very high (hyperthyroidism) secretion of hormones by thyroid gland. You therefore exhibit symptoms of hypothyroidism like weight gain, intolerance to cold, nervousness, and others. You could also exhibit symptoms of hyperthyroidism like weight loss, heat intolerance, and increased appetite. However, such symptoms are difficult to diagnose, as they are not specific. If you suffer from multi-nodular goiter, your blood pressure and palpitations increase. You are unable to sleep peacefully.

===\\\===\\\===\\\===\\\===\\\===\\\===

24. Complications of Thyroid Problems

Thyroid disorders can be easily managed if detected and treated early. Serious complications then occur only rarely. However, if left undiagnosed or not treated properly, serious complications ensue and sometimes turn fatal.

Thyroid Disorder Complications

Thyroid disorders lead to various health problems if unattended. These include:

Heart Ailments

Hypothyroidism causes low levels of thyroid hormones. This pushes up levels of low-density lipoprotein (LDL) cholesterol in blood. Even subclinical hypothyroidism, a mild form of hypothyroidism, can push cholesterol levels excessively. High cholesterol in blood hampers heart pumping. Sometimes it enlarges your heart and consequently causes heart failure.

Goiter

Pituitary gland secretes more TSH or thyroid-stimulating hormone to instigate thyroid gland to produce more hormones. Constant stimulation forces thyroid gland to enlarge leading to goiter. An enlarged thyroid gland not only affects your appearance but also poses problems in breathing and swallowing.

Peripheral Neuropathy

Nerves carry information from brain to different body parts. These are peripheral nerves. Latent hypothyroidism undiagnosed and untreated damages these nerves. This causes numbness, pain, and a tingling sensation in your arms. At times, it causes loss of muscle control.

Myxedema

Prolonged and undiagnosed hypothyroidism could eventually lead to Myxedema. This is a rare medical condition. You develop intense intolerance to cold. You feel drowsy and lazy all day long. You lose consciousness often. You could also slip into coma. This requires immediate medical treatment. If you develop infection or stress of any kind, complications compound further.

Depression

Continuous hypothyroidism if left untreated becomes severe over time. It slows down normal brain functioning. This translates into depression and poor mental health.

Birth Defects

Children born to women with untreated thyroid problems could develop serious complications. These complications could be present at the time of birth or develop later in life. Often such children face serious mental and physical health problems. However, most complications can be treated if diagnosed and treated early.

Infertility

Hypothyroidism or low levels of thyroid hormone affect fertility in women. It upsets regular ovulation process. You require fertility enhancement medications or hormone replacement therapy.

Thyroid Storm

Sometimes hypothyroidism leads to severe life-threatening condition with high fever, high blood pressure, irregular heartbeat, mental confusion, weakness, restlessness, and even enlargement of liver. This extreme condition is thyroid storm. It could induce coma and sometimes it turns fatal.

Suppurative Thyroiditis

This is a rare medical condition causing infection of thyroid gland. Thyroid is normally infection resistant. However, thyroid disorders weaken the gland and it becomes susceptible to infections. If you already have Hashimoto's thyroiditis, you are at a greater risk of developing suppurative thyroiditis. This starts as an upper respiratory tract infection and symptoms include neck pain, fever, rash, and difficulty in talking and swallowing.

Obesity

Thyroid disorders make you obese. Obesity causes serious health problems like heart ailments, excessive fatigue, pain in joints, and various others.

High Blood Pressure

Blood pressure is the force of blood against artery walls when your heart beats. Normal blood pressure should be 120 over 80 mmHg. Blood pressure is not the same always. Hypothyroidism lowers heart rate to less than 60 beats per minute due to poor pumping pressure of heart. Blood vessel walls stiffen. Hyperthyroidism pushes heart beat rate to very high levels. Heart pumps blood vigorously. This weakens your heart and arteries are unable to withstand the force of blood against the walls. Arteries rupture and eventually cause heart failure.

===\\\===\\\===\\\===\\\===\\\===\\\===

25. Ten Warning Signs of Thyroid Problems

Thyroid gland functions affect every part of your body. Your mental and physical health is governed by thyroid hormones. Misbalance in hormone levels affects your health adversely. Often, you are unable to understand thyroid disorder symptoms. Left undiagnosed, these symptoms manifest into serious medical problems like heart ailments, obesity, infertility, depression, and similar others.

Often thyroid problems remain undetected. Majority of people with thyroid are unaware of it. Remain aware of the warning signs that indicate thyroid problems:

1. Exhaustion and Tiredness: You feel tired and fatigued always even after sleeping soundly at night. You require frequent naps. If you have hyperthyroidism, you are unable to sleep and hence are tired and exhausted.

2. Weight Changes: Despite eating a healthy diet and exercising regularly, you are unable to shed weight. Or else, you are constantly losing weight despite eating the same diet and maintaining regular exercises. Excessive weight gain or loss indicates thyroid disorders. Excess secretion of thyroid hormones or hyperthyroidism burns body energy faster. You lose considerable weight despite having an increased appetite and consuming more food. Low secretion of thyroid hormones or hypothyroidism lowers metabolic rate. Less energy is consumed and you gain weight despite having a controlled diet and exercising. Constipation sets in, as digestion is slow and delayed.

3. Nervous Disorders: Panic attacks or feeling extremely anxious is due to hyperthyroidism. If you feel sad and depressed for no specific reason, it could be due to hypothyroidism. Antidepressants do not provide any relief.

4. Cholesterol Levels: Thyroid disorders disrupt blood cholesterol levels. Undiagnosed hypothyroidism increases cholesterol levels while hyperthyroidism lowers blood cholesterol levels. Medications do not cause any change at all.

5. Family History: If your family members suffer from thyroid disorders, there is every chance of you developing such disorders sometime in your life. Often mild thyroid disorders remain undetected. However, you may develop a distinct thyroid problem.

6. Menstrual Irregularities: Irregular periods, heavy or scanty periods, and sometimes, painful periods are an indication of thyroid disorders. Undiagnosed thyroid problems could lead to infertility.

7. Bowel Movements: Severe constipation is often due to hypothyroidism while frequent diarrhea is due to hyperthyroidism. Sudden changes in bowel movements also indicate thyroid disorders.

8. Changes in Skin and Hair: Thyroid disorders make hair brittle and coarse. Hair loss is high. Your skin becomes dry, scaly, and thick. Hyperthyroidism makes your skin thin and fragile. Hypothyroidism leads to hair loss along edge of eyebrow.

9. Enlargement of Neck: Swelling of neck, voice turning hoarse, and difficulty in swallowing or breathing indicate thyroid problems.

10. Tendonitis and Muscular Problems: Muscular pains, joint pains, weakness in arms and legs indicate thyroid problems.

I advise you to seek medical advice to overcome these problems, as timely medical help can provide remedial measures.

===\\\===\\\===\\\===\\\===\\\===\\\===

26. The Unhealthy Thyroid - Is Your Thyroid Making You Sick and Tired?

Your thyroid is a small butterfly-shaped gland in the neck. When it functions normally, you are hardly aware of its existence. However, a small malfunction of this gland causes extensive changes in your health and disturbs your regular routine.

Thyroid and You

When hormone secretion by thyroid gland is in excess or less than normal levels your body displays various symptoms like fatigue, weight changes, anxiety, dry skin, irregular menstrual periods, hair fall, and various others. Often, you ignore or dismiss these symptoms. You feel symptoms are due to irregular eating habits, stress, advancing age, and similar others.

Most thyroid symptoms are same as those of various ailments or age-related problems like menopause, arthritis, depression, anxiety, nervous disorders, panic issues, diabetes, irritable bowel syndrome, and others. Further, a swollen neck alone does not indicate thyroid disease. The best way to determine thyroid disorder is through a blood test.

Thyroid gland affects every single part of your body as hormones produced by this gland are circulated throughout your body through blood. Hence, if your thyroid gland falls sick or becomes unhealthy, it affects your entire physical and mental existence. Nonetheless, almost all problems occurring due to thyroid gland can be overcome easily and effectively. Early diagnosis coupled with prompt and regular treatment cures most thyroid disorders.

Major Thyroid Disorders

Depression and Anxiety

This is a serious disorder of nervous system. Yet, if you have hyperthyroidism, you develop severe mood swings and often suffer from depression, panic attacks, anxiety pangs, fear, erratic behavior, and similar mental ailments. Symptoms point singularly towards mental problems. Nonetheless, a thyroid check-up could reveal hyperthyroidism. Treating this would help restore your mental health.

Cholesterol Levels in Blood

Hypothyroidism increases cholesterol levels in blood. Very high cholesterol could lead to heart ailments and sometimes, even heart failure. Cholesterol can be detected only through a blood test. If it shows high levels, I suggest you go for a thyroid check-up. If it shows hypothyroidism, treating it would reduce your cholesterol levels in blood.

Menopause

Irregular periods or scanty periods are common during perimenopause and menopause. Hormonal changes during this period bring about major changes in your physical appearance and mental health like weight gain, mood swings, anxiety, and many others. Most such symptoms are common to thyroid disorders. Only a blood test and thyroid check-up can clearly diagnose your actual medical condition.

Heart Ailments

Hypothyroidism causes slow heartbeat rates. Hyperthyroidism causes fast heartbeat rates. Both cause heart problems. High cholesterol levels in blood increase such symptoms. Often, an overactive thyroid gland cause abnormal heart rhythms leading to sudden blood clotting and consequent stroke. Most of these symptoms are common in people with heart ailments. If thyroid disorder remains undiagnosed in such conditions, it leads to serious problems.

===\\\===\\\===\\\===\\\===\\\===\\\===

27. What to Expect When Someone has a Thyroid Disease?

Thyroid disorders are a common medical problem in the United States. Millions of women have hypothyroidism and often many remain undiagnosed. Many elderly men also exhibit thyroid disorder symptoms. These symptoms have a serious and long-term effect on your mental and physical health. Prolonged and undiagnosed symptoms of thyroid disorder eventually cause multifarious health issues.

Symptoms of thyroid disease are similar to various other health problems. Rather, they often overlap symptoms of postpartum period, premenstrual hormonal changes, menopause, depression, stress, heart ailments, and many others.

Thyroid Problem Indicators

Although some of these symptoms seem ambiguous, if you suffer from most of them, it indicates a thyroid imbalance. Common indicators of thyroid problems are:

□ Overtly exhausted and fatigued
□ Unexplained weight loss or gain
□ Depression, panicky, and anxious
□ Extremely irritated and impatient
□ Severe changes in skin and hair like hair thinning, loss of hair, dry and itchy skin, moist and thin skin
□ Extreme intolerance to heat or cold
□ Severe mood swings

▫ Disturbed and changing sleep patterns
▫ Disinterested in life

Why thyroid symptoms remain undiagnosed?

Tiredness, stress, anxiety, and depression are common symptoms. Often serious problems in life like divorce, death of a loved one, loss of job, and various personal happenings are stressful and you feel depressed over the outcome of these happenings. Excessive workload causes fatigue. Further, most thyroid symptoms are subtle and do not manifest fully in the early stages.

Women in perimenopause and menopause also experience similar symptoms. Sometimes physical symptoms like a rapid heartbeat indicate heart problems. However, it is also a symptom of hyperthyroidism. Gynecological problems are attributed to hormonal changes occurring in a woman's body as she undergoes different phases of her life like childbirth, post partum, perimenopause, menopause, and others.

Further, you do not disclose most symptoms in detail to your doctor. You feel your excessive workload is the root cause for all physical and mental problems. Medications for stress and anxiety do not deliver desired results. Change of medicines only prolongs the problem.

===\\\===\\\===\\\===\\\===\\\===\\\===

28. Genetics of Thyroid Problems

Thyroid problems -hypothyroidism and hyperthyroidism - occur mainly due to abnormal secretion of thyroid hormones. Autoimmune diseases like Graves' disease and Hashimoto thyroiditis lead to thyroid disorders of hyperthyroidism and hypothyroidism respectively. However, it is not any unwritten rule that people with these diseases are sure to develop thyroid disorders or people with thyroid problems are sure to develop similar autoimmune diseases. Nonetheless, these diseases provide a deep insight into a co-existing relation between genetics and thyroid disorders.

Genetics of Hypothyroidism

Hypothyroidism is when your thyroid gland does not secrete sufficient hormones. Iodine deficiency is considered the major cause for this deficiency. Presently, requisite iodine is available through food. Therefore, primary cause for thyroid problems boils down to genetics.

Congenital hypothyroidism occurs at birth and is due to either an inactive or a deformed thyroid gland. Numerous genes are responsible for formation of thyroid gland while baby is in womb, and thereafter, to secrete thyroid hormones in the gland. If any of these genes malfunction due to any reason, thyroid gland may not form properly or may not secrete hormones normally.

Another genetic link is to have the correct number of chromosomes. If you suffer from syndromes, number of chromosomes in your genes is incorrect. This causes thyroid disorders. Your body immune system functions through genes. If you suffer from any autoimmune disorder, antibodies affect your own body tissue. Thyroid disorders are also due to autoimmune diseases.

If genetics are the primary cause for thyroid disorders, then every member of a family with thyroid disorder should develop it sometime or the other. However, it is not so. Some people with strong family history of thyroid problems do not pass it on to other family members while some with almost very minimal family history continue to have it across each generation. Hence, you cannot conclude that genes are responsible for thyroid disorders.

The best way to tackle thyroid disorders is to have regular medical check-ups. Check your thyroid levels after pregnancy. Women over the age of fifty should undergo thyroid check-ups regularly.

===\\\===\\\===\\\===\\\===\\\===\\\===

29. Thyroid Disorders and Diabetes

Thyroid problems and diabetes are both endocrine disorders. If you have diabetes, you are at a greater risk of developing thyroid disorders. Thyroid problems could be either hypothyroidism or hyperthyroidism. Hypothyroidism lowers metabolism rates while hyperthyroidism increases metabolism rates.

Thyroid disorders are often due to autoimmune diseases. Type I diabetes is also an autoimmune disorder. Hence, if you have a type of autoimmune disorder, chances of you developing another one is much higher than people with no autoimmune disorders.

Hypothyroidism and Diabetes

Hypothyroidism lowers metabolism rates. Blood flow is slower. Diabetes medications keep circulating in your blood for a longer time. Therefore, glucose levels in blood drop. I would advise you to reduce dosage of diabetes medications to control glucose levels from dropping very low.

Hyperthyroidism and Diabetes

Hyperthyroidism increases metabolism rates. Blood flow is faster. Diabetes medications do not remain in circulation in your blood for a long time. Therefore, glucose levels in blood shoot up. You need more insulin. Higher thyroid hormone production pushes glucose secretion in liver and it is absorbed very fast in your intestines. Insulin resistance increases. You start sweating and develop tremors. These symptoms are common to diabetic and hyperthyroidism patients. Being diabetic, you feel your glucose levels have dropped too much and you eat. This pushes your blood glucose levels further. I would advise you to verify glucose levels with a glucose meter and thereafter take necessary medicines or eat food.

Hyperthyroidism increases heart rate. Sometimes heart beat rhythm is abnormal. This causes chest pain. In extreme cases, this causes further deterioration of heart problems and could lead to heart failure.

Untreated hyperthyroidism is responsible for thinning of bones leading to osteoporosis. Diabetic people often suffer from stimuli loss and as a result are unsure of their steps. Hence, a combination of hyperthyroidism and diabetes makes you prone to bone injuries, especially in the elderly.

Pregnancy, Diabetes, and Thyroid Disorders

Postpartum thyroiditis is a form of autoimmune thyroid disease affecting women within the first year of childbirth. Diabetic women are at a greater risk of developing it than normal women. Normal thyroid functions and blood glucose levels should be carefully monitored and controlled in pregnant women.

===\\\===\\\===\\\===\\\===\\\===\\\===

30. Thyroid Conditions and Hormones

Thyroid gland produces hormones that influence major body processes. These hormones are responsible for body growth, development, metabolism, sexual function, reproduction, and your mental health. When thyroid hormone secretion is insufficient, rate of energy usage is low. This leads to hypothyroidism. When thyroid hormones are produced in excess, rate of energy usage increases. This leads to hyperthyroidism.

Thyroid Hormones and Thyroid Conditions

Thyroid hormone or TH is the only major biochemical molecule to incorporate iodine. TH exists in two forms:

1. Thyroxin or T4
2. Triiodothyronine or T3

T4 is an inactive form and has to be converted into T3 to become active. T3 is eight times more effective than T4. Conversion of T4 into T3 takes place in thyroid, liver, brain, blood, and various body tissues. TH is sensitive to other body hormones. Estrogen found in women reduces efficiency of TH. Hence, women produce more thyroid hormones than men do. Women are also more prone to thyroid disorders than men are.

TH Imbalance and Hypothyroidism

TH imbalance affects your mental health extensively. T3 influences serotonin levels. Low T3 levels lead to depression. Hypothyroid people suffer from mental confusion, turn paranoid, suffer memory loss, and often hallucinate. These symptoms aggravate with age. Other symptoms of hypothyroid include extensive fatigue and tiredness. All together cause stress and depression.

Low TH levels in blood are also responsible for low blood sugar, slow digestion, and constipation. Low TH levels also lead to infertility. TH helps control heart rate and blood pressure. TH imbalance leads to very slow heartbeat rate and blood pressure could fall to as low as 70/50. Breathing is difficult. Muscular pains increase. When TH levels drop, liver is unable to function normally and produces excess cholesterol, triglycerides, and fatty acids. This increases heart risks.

TH Imbalance and Hyperthyroidism

Hyperthyroidism increases heartbeat rate. You are unable to sleep and become irritated and tired. High TH levels pep your energy levels extensively such that you behave like a maniac. You experience tremors. You are more prone to thyroid storms, which could eventually translate into heart failure and death.

===\\\===\\\===\\\===\\\===\\\===\\\===

31. Thyroid Problems in Women

Common thyroid problems in women include hypothyroidism and hyperthyroidism.

Hypothyroidism: Thyroid gland produces insufficient amounts of thyroid hormones – T3 and T4 – leading to hypothyroidism. Women with hypothyroidism do not ovulate normally and hence have problems in conceiving. It is difficult to diagnose thyroid problems in pregnant women. Yet it is important as undiagnosed thyroid problems could lead to growth retardation of fetus, stillbirth, anemia, and others.

Symptoms of hypothyroidism in women include:

□ Weight gain
□ Persistent tiredness
□ Lethargy
□ Intolerance to cold
□ Dry puffy skin
□ Constipation
□ Swollen joints
□ Heavy menstrual periods
□ High cholesterol levels
□ Muscular pain
□ Brittle fingernails
□ Hoarseness in voice
□ Depression

Hyperthyroidism: Thyroid gland produces excessive thyroid hormones causing hyperthyroidism. Symptoms of hyperthyroidism in women include:

▫ Weight loss
▫ Fatigue
▫ Intolerance to heat
▫ Fast Heartbeat
▫ Frequent bowel movements
▫ Irregular and scanty menstruation
▫ Muscular weakness
▫ Insomnia

Other Thyroid Problems

Post Pregnancy

A minor percentage of women suffer from thyroid problems after giving birth to baby. Your thyroid gland swells and hormone production is disturbed. It could be either hypothyroidism or hyperthyroidism. I prescribe medications accordingly. Normally, such thyroid disorders settle down with a year of childbirth.

Thyroid Cancer

This thyroid disorders occurs rarely. There is no specific cause for its occurrence. Many hint that radiation therapy treatments on neck and head could eventually lead to thyroid cancer. Radiation treatment involves focusing of light and heat. These harm thyroid gland and possibility of cancer increases.

Thyroid Nodules

One or many nodules form within thyroid gland causing swelling of gland. These nodules are lumps. Most lumps contain fluid while some are solid lumps. These lumps impair normal thyroid functioning often leading to hyperthyroidism. Sometimes these nodules become very large and cause problems in swallowing and breathing. You cough frequently and voice turns hoarse. Excessive intake of goitrogenic foods leads to formation of thyroid nodules.

Inactive Thyroid

Sometimes it becomes necessary to remove a part or major part of your thyroid gland. This causes various thyroid disorders in women like irregularities in menstrual cycles, heavy menstrual bleeding, pain during menstruation, and others.

Autoimmune Disorders

Thyroid dysfunction causes autoimmune disorders like Hashimoto's thyroiditis and Graves' disease. Immune system repels and antibodies attack your own body tissue. Thyroid gland swells and is unable to sustain that attack. Hormone production is affected as thyroid function is severely disrupted.

Most thyroid problems can be treated. Medications, treatments, or surgery for thyroid disorders in women depends on the severity of symptoms and your normal health. If you have various other ailments, thyroid disorder treatment should be in conjunction with treatment for other ailments. If thyroid gland is removed, you need hormone replacements for life.

===\\\===\\\===\\\===\\\===\\\===\\\===

32. Thyroid Disease and Pregnancy

Women with thyroid problems in the past have a greater risk of developing them again during pregnancy. Otherwise, only a minor percentage of women suffer thyroid disorders during pregnancy. It is best to normalize thyroid functions before conception in women with thyroid disorders.

Hormonal Changes and Thyroid

Estrogen and gonadotropin hormones present in pregnant women increase thyroid hormone levels in blood. Gonadotropin is similar to TSH and hence stimulates thyroid to produce more hormones. Higher levels of estrogen in blood produce higher levels of globulin protein. This protein transports thyroid hormone in blood.

It is difficult to detect thyroid disorders during pregnancy due to such hormonal changes. Thyroid gland enlarges a little during pregnancy. Noticeably enlarged thyroid in pregnant women should be immediately evaluated as it could indicate thyroid disease. Further, thyroid disorder symptoms like fatigue, weight gain, mood swings, and others are common to both pregnancy and thyroid disorders. Hence diagnosis is little difficult.

Hyperthyroidism and Pregnancy

Hyperthyroidism in pregnancy is due to autoimmune disorder Graves' disease. Your immune system develops an antibody, thyroid-stimulating immunoglobulin, or TSI. This stimulates excess hormone secretion. If you already have Graves' disease and are pregnant, you find an improvement in most symptoms of Graves' disease in second and third trimesters. Further, most symptoms are suppressed in the final term of pregnancy. However, you experience worsening symptoms of Graves' disease within the first few months of delivery. It subsequently relapses in the postpartum. Hence, you require careful monitoring of symptoms and treatment during your pregnancy.

Uncontrolled hyperthyroidism during pregnancy has several far-reaching effects. It leads to preeclampsia or a sudden increase in blood pressure in late pregnancy, premature birth, congestive heart failure, miscarriage, low birth weight, and thyroid storm.

Hyperthyroidism in a newborn leads to low weight, increases heart rate leading to heart failure, early closure of soft spot in skull, an enlarged thyroid leading to problems in breathing. If you have had radioactive iodine treatment in the past for Graves' disease, antibodies could still be present even with normal thyroid levels. These antibodies stimulate fetal thyroid. However, baby may not develop hyperthyroidism if mother is on anti-thyroid medications.

Mild hyperthyroidism during pregnancy does not require any treatment. I would not advise radioactive iodine treatment for pregnant women. I would suggest lowest possible dosages of anti-thyroid medications as it travels through placenta and could decrease fetal thyroid hormone production leading to hypothyroidism. Mothers on moderate anti-thyroid medications can breastfeed. Preferably, doses should be taken after feedings and infants should be regularly monitored.

Hypothyroidism and Pregnancy

Hashimoto's disease leads to hypothyroidism in pregnancy. This autoimmune disease affects hormone production in thyroid gland. Inflammation of gland lowers hormone secretion. Hypothyroidism in pregnancy often results from inadequately treated hypothyroidism in the past or from removal or destruction of thyroid gland.

Uncontrolled hypothyroidism in the first trimester affects nervous system and brain development in fetus. Later, it could cause stillbirth, anemia, miscarriage, low birth weight, preeclampsia, or a sudden increase in blood pressure in late pregnancy, and in rare cases, congestive heart failure.

Hypothyroidism in pregnant women is treated with synthetic thyroid hormone or thyroxin. This is a safe medication for pregnant women. If subclinical hypothyroidism is discovered during pregnancy, I would suggest appropriate treatment to ensure a healthy pregnancy since the condition is associated with maternal and fetal complications. If you already have hypothyroidism and are now pregnant, you should increase dosage to maintain normal levels of thyroid hormone. I would advise checking of thyroid functions once in two months.

===\\\===\\\===\\\===\\\===\\\===\\\===

33. Thyroid Problems in Children

Thyroid disorders are possible in infants and children. However, rate of incidence is much lower than those of adults are. Thyroid problems in children could be congenital hypothyroidism, Hashimoto's thyroiditis, Graves' disease, and others.

Thyroid disorders in children should be diagnosed early. Appropriate treatments should also be started early. Thyroid dysfunction not only disrupts your child's growth; it could also lead to serious complications later in life. Rather, it would then not be possible to treat such complications.

Symptoms of Thyroid Disorders

Infants
▫ Prolonged jaundice: Jaundice is normal in newborns. However, prolonged jaundice symptoms indicate poor thyroid functions.
▫ Huge soft spots on skull
▫ Constipation
▫ Poor feeding
▫ Excessive sleep
▫ Less crying

Younger Children
▫ Puffy face with protruding eyes due to Graves's disease
▫ Improper growth
▫ Delayed growth of teeth
▫ Short stature
▫ Overweight
▫ Thin hair

▫ Dry skin

Older Children
▫ Fatigue
▫ Excessive intolerance to cold
▫ Slow heartbeat
▫ Attention deficiency
▫ Poor memory
▫ Excessive sleep or could also be insomnia
▫ Dry skin

Thyroid Disorders in Children

Congenital Hypothyroidism: This disorder affects one in four thousand babies. It occurs due to poor thyroid gland formation or complete absence of thyroid gland. This should be diagnosed very early; otherwise, it could lead to severe mental retardation and various growth and developmental problems. Newborns are tested for thyroid functions in the first week of their birth. If diagnosis hints at congenital hypothyroidism, thyroid hormone replacement therapy is immediately administered.

Hyperthyroidism in Newborns: This is neonatal hyperthyroidism. If mother has Graves's disease, thyroid-stimulating antibodies stimulate thyroid gland of fetus. Thyroid hormones are in excess. If such antibodies clear off within two to three months, I do not advise any treatment. However, if they cause thyrotoxicosis, immediate anti-thyroid treatment is necessary to correct hormonal imbalance.

Hashimoto's Thyroiditis: This is the primary cause for hypothyroidism in children. Since symptoms evolve gradually, often they remain undiagnosed. As thyroid gland remains inactive, physical and mental changes are clearly seen. I advise a daily dosage of thyroid hormone replacement according to age. Most symptoms soon disappear.

However, behavioral problems arise as mental and physical processes boost with such medications. Regular monitoring can absolve all such problems.

Graves' Disease: This is the primary cause for hyperthyroidism in children. Antibodies increase thyroid hormone secretion. The most prominent symptom is increased energy levels, being hyperactive, restless, and being noisier than other children. Overall, academic performance is poor as their concentration levels are very low. A blood test can detect levels of thyroid stimulating hormone and thyroid hormones in blood. I advise starting of appropriate treatment immediately. Anti-thyroid drugs like carbimazole and propylthiouracil can stabilize condition. In severe cases, radioactive iodine or surgery is essential. Side effects of medications include mouth ulcers, sore throats, skin rashes, and low count of platelets.

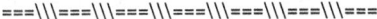

===\\\===\\\===\\\===\\\===\\\===\\\===

34. Thyroid Problems in Elderly

Thyroid problems normally compound in the elderly. Thyroid diseases affect women more than men. Further, it causes serious complications in elderly women in their menopausal years. The elderly should always start with low doses of thyroid medications. Increases should be gradual and slow.

Common Thyroid Disorders Affecting the Elderly

Osteoporosis: It is normal for menopausal women to lose bone strength as they age. As estrogen levels decline in menopausal women, they are more prone to bone injuries and fractures. Some women also develop low bone density or osteoporosis. This disease has no symptoms and you realize it only when you suffer a fracture. It is normal body function for bones to break down and build up by themselves. However, with advancing age and high concentrations of thyroid hormones, this breakdown process accelerates. Bones do not build up by themselves and hence bone loss is excessive.

I suggest proper treatment of hyperthyroidism to lower hormone levels in blood. This would stop bone loss. Include calcium rich foods in your diet and take calcium supplements.

Myxedema Coma: Untreated hypothyroidism slowly progresses towards a fatal condition, myxedema coma. Stress, heart ailments and failure, trauma, severe cold, and certain drugs accelerate the process. Myxedema coma induces sudden fall in body temperature, urine retention, and loss of lung function, constipation, seizures, and disorientation. Soon you pass into a state of coma and in most cases death is the final eventuality.

I advise immediate hospitalization and prompt medical attention to combat myxedema coma.

Heart Disease: Hypothyroidism increases cholesterol levels in blood. Further, an underactive thyroid increases cholesterol absorbed in blood and it is then difficult for liver to eliminate cholesterol. Hypothyroidism also increases blood pressure. Heartbeat rate is low with hypothyroidism. This results in hypertension. Eventually you develop stroke, heart attack, and heart failure. Presence of high levels of cholesterol adds to the risk factor. Hyperthyroidism increases heartbeat rate excessively. If you already have heart ailments, hyperthyroidism compounds it further.

Amiodarone is a specific anti-arrhythmic medication. It is very effective for ventricular arrhythmias as it slows down nerve impulses of heart. However, Amiodarone contains iodine. People with thyroid disorders should avoid this drug, as it is problematic for hypothyroidism and hyperthyroidism.

Thyroid Storm: Elderly people are at a greater risk of thyroid storm. This is a rare medical condition when blood pressure is excessively high. Other simultaneous medical situations include uncontrollable heartbeat rate, severe chest pain, weakness, mood swings, high fever, and shortness of breath, confusion, and extensive sweating. Some people pass into a coma.

This condition requires immediate medical help. I would advise high doses of anti-thyroid medications, iodine-containing compounds, and thereafter, necessary therapy to treat specific underlying medical problems. If you also suffer from emotional stress, infections, or regular changes in blood sugar levels, thyroid storm is almost a certainty.

===\\\===\\\===\\\===\\\===\\\===\\\===

Part-III: Tests and Diagnosis for Thyroid Diseases

35. Importance of Early Diagnosis of Your Thyroid Problems

Thyroid gland is one of the endocrine glands of your body. Thyroid hormone, thyroxin, is responsible for important body functions like mental health, physical growth, control of body temperature, and others. Thyroxin should be at correct levels in your body. Only then, all body functions can be normal. When thyroid hormone levels in body is low, it is hypothyroidism, and when hormone levels are high, it is hyperthyroidism.

Diagnosis of Thyroid Problems

Thyroid disorders develop over a long period spreading across months and years. Symptoms are subtle at first and later, they become prominent. Thyroid problems affect men, women, and children, although the incidence is highest among women. Sometimes elderly men are affected.

Children

In children, thyroid problems could be present at birth or may appear later in childhood as well. A newborn baby could be born without a thyroid gland or with a partially functioning gland. This is congenital thyroidism. Some babies develop hypothyroidism in infancy, although it is difficult to detect. Symptoms include:

▫ Prolonged jaundice
▫ Protruding tongue
▫ Constipation

- Feeding difficulties
- Cold hands and feet
- Puffy face
- Hoarse cry
- Umbilical hernia
- Speckled skin
- Soft skull

Importance of Early diagnosis

Affected babies seem normal at birth. However, symptoms erupt soon thereafter. Some children develop thyroid disorders much later. These disorders could be inherited or develop without genetic linkage. Such children have retarded growth, are inattentive at school, find it difficult to concentrate, feel fatigued all through the day, and register significant weight changes. Sometimes autoimmune disease causes thyroid problems in children. Cells of immune system act against thyroid gland cells thereby inhibiting normal hormone secretion.

Early diagnosis is very important as growth of baby is immediately affected. This translates into poor brain development, lack of growth of motor skills, poor language, and reading abilities, and attention disorders. Child with thyroid problems should be carefully monitored. Careful evaluation of clinical indications is essential to detect exact nature of thyroid problem so that effective treatment can be carried out. Absence of appropriate treatment or delaying treatment shunts physical and mental growth of your child. Once thyroid disorder is taken care of, body metabolism normalizes and normal growth and development takes place.

Adults and the Elderly

Thyroid disorders may not erupt during pregnancy, as your body immune system remains suppressed to protect growing fetus. However, if you had thyroid problems in the past, it could develop in the initial months after delivery. Nonetheless, you should undergo necessary checks to analyze thyroid condition during pregnancy as problems affect fetus seriously.

Although menopausal women are at a greater risk of developing thyroid disorders, younger women, and men could also develop them. Common symptoms include:

▫ Breathlessness
▫ Intolerance to heat or cold
▫ Muscular pains
▫ Joint pains
▫ Irritability
▫ Disorientation
▫ Irregular heartbeat
▫ Chest pain
▫ Fever

Seek immediate medical attention if you develop such symptoms. Deferring medical attention could lead to serious calamities, sometimes even life threatening. Thyroid disorders and deficiencies affect your brain and heart. Your body immune system weakens and you are unable to bear pain, trauma, or any emotional or physical exertion. Sometimes these disorders translate into cancer.

Early diagnosis helps you overcome thyroid problems. Symptoms manifest gradually and often you are unable to recognize or pinpoint symptoms. Sometimes other ailments like heart diseases, blood pressure problems, menopause, and normal aging problems camouflage thyroid disorder symptoms. You can maintain an active life even if you are on thyroid medication. You feel emotionally stable and can withstand any disturbances.

===\\\===\\\===\\\===\\\===\\\===\\\===

102.

36. Diagnosing Thyroid Disease

Thyroid disease diagnosis covers various processes like physical examination, blood tests, imaging tests, biopsies, and others.

Physical Examination

Doctor conducts a thorough physical examination of your neck and throat. Doctor checks gland's size, firmness of thyroid, enlarged lymph nodes in neck and looks for any possible lumps. Examination includes:

Neck Palpating: Doctor examines your neck for nodules, lumps, thyroid enlargement, or any mass around thyroid. This examination can also detect any increased blood flow around thyroid as this causes palpations. Doctor's stethoscope can detect increased blood flow through the sound.

Heart and blood pressure: Doctors check heartbeat rate. A slow heartbeat rate indicates hypothyroidism while a fast heartbeat rate indicates hyperthyroidism. Few hyperthyroidism patients have high blood pressure. Hence checking of blood pressure can detect irregularities like arterial fibrillation, palpitations, and other heart functions.

Reflex Testing: Doctor uses a mallet on knees and Achilles region to check your reflexes. If reflexes are slow, it indicates hypothyroidism while hyper reflexes indicate hyperthyroidism. Doctor also checks for various other symptoms like slow movements, slow speech, shaky hands, body tremors, sudden movements of feet and hands, swelling of hands and feet.

Body Temperature: An underactive thyroid lowers body temperature excessively.

Weight Check: Doctor will check changes related to your weight. Weight gain without dietary changes indicates hyperthyroidism while weight loss indicates hypothyroidism.

Facial Examination: Thyroid disorders cause puffiness of face, swelling of eyelids, loss of hair in outer edge of eyebrows, and others. Doctor checks your face thoroughly to locate such symptoms of thyroid problems. Doctor checks your soles and palms for presence of carotene. This is an orange-colored deposit occurring due to thyroid disorders.

Skin Examination: Thyroid causes various changes in skin quality. Doctor examines your skin for rough patches in between, excessively smooth skin, yellowish color of skin, or blisters and bumps on forehead.

Hair Examination: Coarse and brittle hair indicates hypothyroidism while fine and thinning hair indicates hyperthyroidism. Hair loss is predominant in both.

Eye Examination: Thyroid disorders affect eyes. Symptoms include protruding eyes, retraction of upper eyelids, constant stare or gaze, infrequent blinking, and uncoordinated movements of upper eyelid. Eyelid does not follow downward movements of eye when you look downwards.

Examination of hands and nails: Doctor checks your hands for any rough patches. Thyroid disorders lead to swollen fingertips. Sometimes nail separates from nail bed causing Plummer's nails.

Diagnostic Tests for Thyroid

Blood Test: Your blood is tested to detect TSH levels. Other blood tests include:

□ Total T4 or Total Thyroxin: Low T4 levels with high TSH indicate hypothyroidism.
□ Total T3 or Total Triiodothyronine: Low T3 with high TSH indicates hypothyroidism.
□ Free T4 or Free Thyroxin: A low free T4 level with high TSH indicates hypothyroidism.
□ Free T3 or Free Triiodothyronine: Low free T3 levels with high TSH indicate hypothyroidism.

Radioactive Iodine Update (RAI-U) Test: This test helps diagnose hyperthyroidism and whether it is due to Graves' disease. It checks ability of thyroid gland to absorb iodine. You drink liquid containing radioactive iodine. An X-ray of thyroid gland soon thereafter shows whether large amounts of iodine settle in your thyroid gland or not. It also detects nodule activity within gland.

Bone Resorption Assessment Test: This is a simple test to detect current rate of bone loss as hyperthyroidism causes serious bone loss. It also detects any other latent bone diseases. This test displays bone strength to support bone therapies and treatments.

Adrenocortex Stress Profile: This test detects levels of cortisol, DHEA, levels of testosterone, and levels of progesterone. The test analyzes results from saliva samples collected over a single day period. Hormones have to pass through cells of saliva gland before entering saliva and therefore this test detects hormone activity levels actually working at cell level. Blood test does not detect actual hormone levels as it measures both available and bio-available levels of hormone. Stress and reproductive hormones influence thyroid hormone production largely.

Food Intolerance and Allergy Testing: This test detects your intolerance levels of various foods like milk, vegetables, fruits, nuts, seeds, spices, and meat. Thyroid levels are extensively influenced by your diet. Lifestyle factors dictate stress levels and all together assess thyroid hormone production in your body.

Ultrasound: An ultrasound of your neck can detect any possibility of neck enlargement (as in goiter), presence of nodules, and if they are fluid-filled or solid-filled.

Radioactive Isotope Thyroid Scan: This produces an image of your thyroid gland to detect exact nature of thyroid enlargement. However, pregnant and lactating women should not undergo this test due to possibility of potential damage to growing fetus or baby through breast-feeding.

Needle Biopsy: This test checks if thyroid nodules are cancerous or not. A fine needle is inserted to draw out fluid and cells from nodule. These are tested to detect presence of cancer cells. Sometimes, if test does not deliver exact results, nodules are surgically removed to rule out possibility of cancer.

===\\\===\\\===\\\===\\\===\\\===\\\===

37. Diagnostic Tests and Procedures for Thyroid Disease

Thyroid disorders are often responsible for changes in your energy levels, weight, and other physical and mental abilities. Thyroid, although a small gland in the neck, is extremely powerful. It is responsible for production and regulation of hormones that help regulate major body functions. Thyroxin hormone produced by thyroid gland is essential for smooth functioning of vital organs like heart, liver, brain, and other body systems.

Excess levels, insufficient levels, or absence of thyroxin is the root cause for major ailments with symptoms like high blood pressure, anxiety, fatigue, forgetfulness, weight fluctuations, palpitations, and others. Risk factors like age, gender, and genetic predisposition highlight possibility of thyroid disorders.

Even if you do not exhibit any symptoms of thyroid ailments, it is best to undergo regular screening as you could develop it anytime.

Diagnostic Tests for Thyroid Diseases

Blood Tests

Thyroid disorders are mainly due to either excess production of thyroid hormones (Hyperthyroidism) or insufficient production of thyroid hormones (Hypothyroidism). A simple blood test can detect hormone levels in body and provide information about several hormones related to thyroid function. You get to know results of your blood test within a week.

Blood tests detect levels of:

T3 or Triiodothyronine: A slight fluctuation in T3 levels is normal and does not hint at any major problem. However, constant high levels of T3 are due to hyperthyroidism while perennially low levels of T3 are due to hypothyroidism.

T4 or Thyroxin: T4 level testing helps in correct diagnosis of whether thyroid disorder is due to problems in thyroid gland or pituitary gland.

Excess T4 in blood indicates an overactive thyroid (hyperthyroidism) while low T4 in blood indicates an underactive thyroid (hypothyroidism).

TSH: This is thyroid-stimulating hormone produced by pituitary gland in brain. This gland instructs thyroid gland when to produce thyroid hormones. High levels of TSH in blood indicate poor production of thyroid hormones. This leads to hypothyroidism. Low levels of TSH in blood indicate excess production of thyroid hormones. This leads to hyperthyroidism.

T3 Resin Uptake or T3RU Test: This test measures amount of proteins circulating in blood that bind to T3 and T4 thyroid hormones. High levels indicate hyperthyroidism while low levels indicate hypothyroidism. Although this test provides an indication of thyroid gland functioning, often, results could be affected due to kidney and liver problems.

Thyroid Antibodies: Most thyroid diseases like Graves's disease or Hashimoto thyroiditis are autoimmune diseases. These instigate your body immune system to release proteins or antibodies. These attack your thyroid gland as if it were a foreign tissue. Test reveals if such antibodies are present in blood and accordingly diagnosis of autoimmune disease responsible for thyroid disorders is possible.

Reverse T3: Under high stress, body does not convert T4 into T3, as is the norm. Instead, body conserves energy in the form of an inactive T3. This is known as ReverseT3 or RT3. Blood test can detect this. However, diagnosis of this test is not acceptable everywhere as some believe that body continues to manufacture RT3 instead of active T3. This is responsible for various ailments and syndromes.

Thyroglobulin Antibodies or Antithyroglobulin Antibodies: Blood test can detect levels of these antibodies. High levels indicate hypothyroidism while low levels indicate hyperthyroidism.

Imaging Tests

Often, blood tests indicate presence of thyroid disorder. However, this is insufficient for a clear and exhaustive diagnosis. Hence, certain additional tests are required. These include:

Radioactive Iodine Uptake (RAIU): Thyroid gland uses iodine from blood to produce thyroid hormones. In this test, you swallow a small radioactive iodine pill. Sometimes doctor gives you an iodine injection. Doctor studies images of radioactivity localized around thyroid gland through a scanning machine. If thyroid gland uses lots of iodine from the pill leading to high RAIU reading, it indicates hyperthyroidism. If thyroid gland uses little iodine from the pill leading to low RAIU reading, it indicates hypothyroidism. Pregnant women should avoid this test.

Ultrasound: This test shows images of structural changes within thyroid gland due to presence of cysts or tumors. Test helps determine type, size, and number of nodules within the gland. Test can also detect presence of lymph nodes, any enlargement of parathyroid glands, or whether nodule is a mass of solid tissue or it is a fluid-filled cyst. However, it cannot determine if a nodule or lump is malignant.

Thyroid Biopsy or Fine Needle Aspiration: A thin needle is directly inserted into thyroid nodules or lumps. Few cells are drawn out. These are tested for cancer. Using ultrasound during biopsy ensures needle enters correct point for testing. Evaluation of biopsy results indicates whether thyroid nodule is cancerous or not. Biopsy can also be done through surgical removal of thyroid tissue. Nonetheless, needle aspiration is preferred over surgical biopsy as it is a simple outpatient procedure and does not take much time. Further, it is less expensive and does not leave any scar.

Computerized Axial Tomography (CT) Scan: Sometimes a CT scan is done to diagnose how far a goiter has invaded into trachea. However, this is not a regular test to detect thyroid disorders. This scan cannot detect small thyroid nodules.

MRI or Magnetic Resonance Imaging: This test cannot detect thyroid functioning or indicate whether it is a case of hyperthyroidism or hypothyroidism. However, MRI can deliver clear images of shape and size of thyroid gland. This helps diagnose enlargement. Further, many prefer MRI scan to x-rays and CT scans, as there is no need of contrast dye or radiation rays.

Unconventional Diagnostic Tests of Thyroid Disease

Although these tests detect thyroid disorders, many do not accept or prescribe them. Yet, tests reveal most thyroid dysfunctions accurately.

Iodine Patch Tests: Pure iodine solution is applied as a patch on a small part of your skin. Rapid absorption indicates iodine deficiency or hypothyroidism.

Basal Body Temperature Testing: This involves testing of body temperature early in the morning, even before active movement starts. A basal temperature much below normal body temperature indicates poor thyroid functioning. However, this test is not accepted as the primary diagnosis.

What do Screening Results Indicate?

Clear results showing very high or very low hormone levels are specific indicators of thyroid disorders like hypothyroidism and hyperthyroidism. Sometimes hormone levels remain within acceptable range, yet indicate a disorder. This is because hormone levels have been steadily increasing or decreasing over a period. This is an apparent sign of a potential problem despite there being no indications thereof.

I would suggest a detailed study of all symptoms and blood and imaging test reports to arrive at the correct diagnosis. Often, such situations could suddenly develop into serious consequences.

If tests indicate hypothyroidism, it is best to start with necessary treatment immediately. However, if tests indicate hyperthyroidism, I would advise waiting and monitoring all symptoms, for some more time. Often, thyroid hormone levels settle down and may not cause any problems at all. If you start with hyperthyroidism treatments immediately, you then suffer various side effects.

Thyroid tests are relatively painless and done easily. Early detection and thorough diagnosis can help you adopt necessary treatment options and prevent serious health complications.

===\\\===\\\===\\\===\\\===\\\===\\\===

38. Key Thyroid Function Tests and Interpretation

Thyroid Function Tests

Clinical detection of thyroid disorders is difficult. Thyroid function tests help in easy and correct diagnosis. Measuring TSH levels is essential. High TSH levels with low levels of free T4 indicate hypothyroidism. Similarly, low TSH with high levels of free T4 indicates hyperthyroidism. Presence of antibodies can establish cause of thyroid dysfunction. Further, intake of different medications and drugs for other ailments also influences levels of thyroid hormones. Hence, it is necessary to analyze all available medical conditions, medications, and reports correctly before final diagnosis is done and treatment is prescribed.

Pregnant women with a previous history of Graves' disease should be screened for TSH receptor autoantibodies. High levels of maternal TSH receptor autoantibodies in the mother can lead to neonatal or even fetal hyperthyroidism. TSH receptor autoantibody levels do not always fall even with appropriate treatment. It is best to go for a thorough check-up soon after pregnancy.

Physiology of the Thyroid Gland

Thyroid gland is a butterfly-shaped gland enveloping itself around the trachea in the upper stretch and around thyroid cartilage in the lower stretch. As you age your spine curves, overlying thyroid tissue thickens, and thyroid gland slips further down. This causes palpitation problems in the elderly. Release of TRH or thyroid releasing hormone from hypothalamus gland in brain depends on various factors. Again, TSH from pituitary is released according to TRH. Under normal conditions, TSH shows diurnal variation with baseline value being present from 10-11 PM and decreasing about 10-11 AM. This affects thyroid hormone secretion and conversion of T4 into T3. However, significant variations occur daily although it appears to be cyclic in nature.

Interpretation of Thyroid Function Testing

Blood tests and imaging tests help detect thyroid disorders. Blood test reveals cellular activities in your body. Accordingly, tests are interpreted. Often, test results and symptoms exhibited by you differ largely. Sometimes, medications prescribed according to test results do not provide desired results. Thyroid hormones in bloodstream do not reach proper equilibrium even with extra cellular fluid and cells. Again, body continues to maintain hormone levels in blood despite activities happening within cells. Hence, thyroid function testing interpretation is very important.

Variables Affecting Test Interpretations

Time of Draw: Normally, thyroid tests should be approximately at the same time as their increases or at the lowest point of TSH. It is best to draw blood early in the morning. Concurrent blood tests done at different timings of the day cannot be considered for a suitable interpretation. You should stick to specific time duration. Otherwise, results will vary.

Reference Range: Blood test deliver result according to specific reference range. This range is determined from a wide population base and does not reflect individual groups. Often people with non-thyroid illness are also included within reference population. Hence, results are affected. Sometimes blood test may not diagnose thyroid problem although you exhibit all symptoms. If you interpret results strictly, thyroid disorders may not be detected as hormonal misbalance may be marginal and hence not within stipulated range.

Same Laboratory: It is best to test for thyroid at the same pathological laboratory. Errors and differences in testing can bring in changes in results. Testing methods and techniques remaining constant, variations and interpretations in results will also remain almost same.

Illness: If you are very ill, suffer from severe ailments, or you are starving due to any reasons, TSH secretion is severely affected. Consequently, conversion of T4 into T3 is reduced extensively. Low levels of TSH and T3 presents a confusing situation. A raised TSH with a normal free T4 is interpreted as interference in TSH secretion. In rare occurrences, pituitary TSH-secreting adenoma or thyroid hormone resistance is attributed to a slightly high TSH with raised free T4.

Ideally, reference range should be interpreted carefully. Diagnosis should be based on a broad criteria involving thorough analysis of symptoms, test reports, and physical examination. Medication in small doses should be prescribed and thereafter reactions should be carefully studied. It takes around a month for thyroid equilibrium to be achieved. Hence, medication effect, retests, and overall change in thyroid symptoms should be studied together to arrive at a consensus.

===\\\===\\\===\\\===\\\===\\\===\\\===

39. Clinical Evaluation - Signs and Features of Thyroid Disease

Thyroid disorders like hypothyroidism and hyperthyroidism have specific characteristic symptoms. These are due to increased or decreased levels of thyroid hormones. Further, localized symptoms like gland enlargement, nodules within gland, and similar others indicate specific thyroid ailment. Sometimes nodules could be malignant.

Hyperthyroidism presents typical symptoms like anxiety, weight loss, diarrhea, tremors, muscular weakness, palpitations, heat intolerance, and others. Hypothyroidism present typical symptoms like weight gain, cold intolerance, dry skin, depression, muscle cramps, menstrual changes, and others.

Goiter or thyroid enlargement can occur in hypothyroidism or hyperthyroidism. Thyroid storm is a case of sudden and fatal conglomeration of all thyroid symptoms. Often, such people exhibit very few symptoms. Sometimes even people with normal thyroid levels display symptoms of enlarged thyroid. Similarly, people with abnormal thyroid levels do not exhibit any symptoms at all.

Clinical Appraisal

Analysis of signs and symptoms of thyroid need not follow any specific decorum. It is a comprehensive analysis of symptoms exhibited, symptoms visible, results of medical tests, and family history. Often, differences between findings of medical tests and clinical recordings make thyroid diagnosis a challenging task.

Sometimes, treatment of non-thyroid conditions leads to thyroid problems. Radioactive treatment in head and neck could cause hypothyroidism. Medications for heart ailments lead to thyroid disorders. Thyroid gland enlargement could also occur due to pregnancy or even adolescence.

Ailments related to sympathetic nervous system display similar symptoms as those of a thyrotoxic person. Over activity of sympathetic nervous system causes anxiety, hypertension, nervousness, and increased metabolism among others. These symptoms are also present in a person with thyroid disorders. If thyroid medications are prescribed, it could lead to a medical calamity.

A family history of thyroid ailments is an apparent symptom. This is very clearly seen in people with a history of autoimmune disorders. Certain thyroid cancers also have a genetic element. Hence, if you have a family history of Goiter or Graves' disease, underlying thyroid symptoms may go unnoticed. Rather, pathological findings could indicate thyroid disorders but goiter symptoms overshadow such findings. Ailment remains diagnosed as goiter and medications are prescribed accordingly.

Appropriate Diagnosis

Thyroid function can be attributed to thyroid tissue ability to absorb iodine and similar iodide compounds. Ultrasound, magnetic resonance imaging (MRI) and CT scanning help in easy identification and analysis of thyroid nodules and their nature as to whether they are benign or malignant. Antithyroglobulin test detects autoimmune thyroiditis. Needle aspiration test analyzes nodules and their contents to decipher if they are cancerous.

Thyroid disorders are common and rampant among major population. However, analysis and diagnosis is often overlooked. Most symptoms are attributed to other ailments like those of the heart, nervous system, old age, and others. Further, many get accustomed to most symptoms and perceive them as a regular habit and not as a medical symptom. Many approach medical help only when condition deteriorates.

However, all thyroid symptoms however severe are treatable. There are innumerable medications and appropriate treatment options available. In certain cases, surgery could also provide immediate relief.

Overall symptoms of hyperthyroidism, hypothyroidism, thyroid cancer, and enlargement should never be analyzed in isolation. Diagnosis should be supported with appropriate medical tests, explanations, comparisons, findings, and a conclusive analysis thereof. If there are any contradictory findings, every aspect of symptoms should be analyzed in perspective. Focusing on a single aspect like family history or psychiatric illness cannot reveal facts about the medical condition. Thyroid ailments are normally not life threatening. A treatment plan that dwells on exact findings and analysis can yield desired results.

===\\\===\\\===\\\===\\\===\\\===\\\===

40. Pathophysiology of Thyroid Disease

Thyroid gland produces two important hormones T4 and T3. These hormones are responsible for almost all important body functions ranging from metabolism, brain functions, bone development, and overall health.

Thyroid gland secretes T4 and T3 hormones using iodide as available in your diet. Your body requires 100ug of iodide to produce your daily requirements of hormones. Your iodine consumption is often governed by geographical factors. Normal dietary ingestion of iodide is between 200 and 500 µg each day. Thyroid gland is equipped with special cells. These cells concentrate iodide thirty to forty times the level found in plasma. This ensures adequate amount of essential iodide in your body for thyroid hormone synthesis. Peroxidase enzyme present in thyroid gland oxidizes iodide into iodine. This iodine undergoes various other processes to eventually produce T4 and T3. Your liver, pituitary, and kidney also use iodine to synthesize T3 from T4.

Thyroid stimulating hormone or TSH is produced from thyrotropin in pituitary gland. T3 is biologically the more active thyroid hormone than T4. Overall thyroid gland secretes only twenty percent of total T3 and T4 production in your body. The rest is available through peripheral metabolism.

Thyroid stimulating hormone or TSH is secreted in the pituitary gland. This hormone regulates hormone synthesis, thyroid gland function, and release of thyroid hormones. Thyrotropin-releasing hormone or TRH produced in hypothalamus influences secretion of TSH. Secretion of TSH and TRH depends on amount of circulating T4 and T3 hormones. When T3 and T4 hormone levels are high, TSH levels are low. When T3 and T4 hormone levels are low, TSH levels are high.

TSH binds to a specific membrane receptor on surface of thyroid epithelial cell. Cell is then activated through adenylate cyclase enzyme. This enzyme is in the plasma membrane. Activation increases intracellular cyclic levels of phosphate. This stimulates further reactions leading to secretion and formation of thyroid hormone. T4 and T3 hormones circulate in blood by binding to specific thyroxin binding globulin proteins and albumin. Only a minor percentage of T4 and T3 remain in a free state.

===\\\===\\\===\\\===\\\===\\\===\\\===

41. Clinical Perspectives in the Diagnosis of Thyroid Disease

If you suffer from thyroid disorders, a physical examination alone can detect the actual disorder. Nonetheless, there are numerous tests, which help in determining your disorder clinically. However, it is not simple to interpret results of such clinical findings. Numerous complexities, limitations, and differences in diagnostic accuracy play an important role in such assessment.

The best interpretations of clinical findings remain restricted to three important tools:

1. Blood tests
2. Imaging Techniques
3. Fine Needle Biopsies

Clinical Perceptions and Perspectives

Testing TSH levels in blood is good when you suspect a thyroid disorder. It is a remarkable screening test as negative predictive value is very high and often most results are negative.

However, screening and diagnosis is not the same. It is possible to have high levels of TSH even without hypothyroidism and hyperthyroidism. TSH values alone cannot be the sole determinant of thyroid deficiency or excess.

Hence, the best clinical approach to analyze disorder in a person with abnormal serum TSH concentration and few unrelated symptoms is to delve deeper into available facts about the abnormality. Analyzing severity of the disease and its underlying causes can shed greater light on actual medical problems. It is then easy to devise suitable remedies.

If you suffer from a serious thyroid disorder and are hospitalized, clinical analysis should be done very carefully. Various illnesses other than thyroid disorders and drugs like dopamine and glucocorticoids can change TSH levels to very high or very low. If physical examination shows a normal thyroid gland, serum test to detect free T4 levels can elaborate actual condition. It is best to allow hormones to settle down and test thereafter. In most such cases, there is no thyroid disease in the strict clinical terminology.

If TSH levels are at abnormally high levels, it is necessary to go in for detailed physical examination with specific attention to thyroid gland.

It is also essential to repeat all tests including imaging tests. Often changes in thyroid gland or development of nodules in thyroid gland do not influence thyroid function extensively. If TSH levels are at abnormal levels and thyroid gland has structural problems, it is not possible to conclude about the possibility of thyroid disorder clinically. Treatment should be advised only after a careful evaluation of all available information with reports of imaging and other tests.

Laboratory interpretations are within specified reference range. This range is not the same for men, women, pregnant women, and children. It is important to interpret hormone levels according to specific range you belong. Thyroid diagnostic tests are not always the stipulated yardstick. Everything is to be studied and interpreted in perspective. Every case of thyroid disorder is different and unique. No case should be analyzed in isolation.

===\\\===\\\===\\\===\\\===\\\===\\\===

42. Your Family Medical History and Thyroid-Related Conditions

Thyroid disorder is more of a familial disorder than a genetic disorder. There is no conclusive evidence that links thyroid disorder to genes. However, thyroid disorders in close relatives like parents, grandparents, children, or siblings influences other family members extensively. Often, in such cases, thyroid diseases develop at a very young age itself.

There are different types of thyroid disorders or thyroiditis. Although thyroid diseases affect close family relations, it is not necessary that they develop the same thyroid disorder. It could be different. Sometimes, thyroid cancer is due to close family linkage of thyroid problems. Nonetheless, there are few thyroid disorders, which follow down the lineage.

Irrespective of such correlations, it is important to undergo thyroid screening regularly. If many family members suffer from thyroid diseases, it is best to check children for any symptoms early in life.

Another connection between thyroid diseases and family history is presence of autoimmune diseases like rheumatoid arthritis in any family member or relations, alive or dead. If any family member suffers from glandular problems like goiter or weight problems, it indicates a possibility of thyroid disease. You stand a higher risk of developing thyroid disorder sometime in your life.

Family here does not refer to your parents or siblings alone. It also includes your aunts, uncles, nephews, nieces, and sometimes your first cousins are included within the definition of your family medical history.

===\\\===\\\===\\\===\\\===\\\===\\\===

43. Clinical Trials and Research Studies on Thyroid Disease

A clinical trial is a scientific experiment. People volunteers participate in clinical trial of medications and dosage. The main purpose of a clinical trial is to assess effectiveness and safety of specific medical devices and best dosage of drugs. Devices and drugs are used on people with specific disease or health condition. Drugs are normally new drugs that have been devised and hence should be tested before being made available to the general population.

Clinical Trials

There are various stages of approval of clinical trials. The first phase spreads over many months. Volunteers are given drugs. Drug reaction is studied in detail as to how it is absorbed, metabolized, and excreted. Dosage levels are increased and thereafter, volunteer reaction is studied to detect side effects.

In the second level of testing spread over around two years, effectiveness of specific drug or device is studied in depth. These are randomized trials. Volunteers are divided into specific groups. One group receives standard treatment while another group receives an experimental drug. Further, neither volunteers nor researchers are aware of who has been given which drug. This helps in delivering a comparative study report about efficacy of specific drug or device. Side effects are clearly discussed and studied.

In the next phase, trial is extended across many thousands of patients. Rather, testing is done on a huge scale and hence spreads over many years. This testing provides extensive understanding of effectiveness of drug. Once this phase is completed successfully, a pharmaceutical company can seek FDA approval to market the drug.

Once you receive FDA approval for consumer sale of specific drug, you need to carry out another survey trial. The main purpose of this trial is to compare new drug with those existing in the market, check and monitor its effectiveness in comparison to other drugs, look how it affects patient's life, and determine cost-effectiveness of drug when compared to other available drugs and therapies. Rather results of this phase are very important and decide whether drug can be circulated in the market or not.

Research Studies

Thyroid disorders like autoimmune diseases and effect of antibodies on thyroid disorders is being researched extensively. Such research is being conducted on mice. Preliminary reports indicate that it is possible to detect autoimmune disease at its root thereby restricting its ability to lead to thyroid disorders. However, adequate medical information is not yet available.

Thyroid gland functions are still not clearly elaborated and evaluated in detail. Thyroid hormone function, pathology of thyroid disease, and how it affects body parts in human is not clear. It is essential to understand which function leads to another. Since researchers have not yet been able to provide any elaborate guidelines on this, thyroid disorders continue to be rampant.

===\\\===\\\===\\\===\\\===\\\===\\\===

Part-IV: Treatments and Medications for Thyroid Diseases

44. Evaluating Your Thyroid Disease Risk

Thyroid disorders cannot be prevented. Nonetheless, early detection assures speedy recovery, fewer complications, and early return to normalcy.

Thyroid disorders could certainly occur in certain persons while it does not or rather may not occur in others.

Evaluating Your Chances of Thyroid Disease

If you fall into any of the following categories, your chances of developing thyroid diseases are high. These risk factors include:

Gender: Women are a high risk of developing thyroid disease than men. Women are eight times more susceptible to thyroid disorders than men are.

Family History: If your parents, siblings, grandparents, aunts, uncles, first cousins, or children have thyroid disorders or have had it in the past, you could develop thyroid problems. Further, familial connections are not necessarily among those who are alive. It could also connect to family relations who have already died.

Age: Normally elderly people have a higher risk of developing thyroid disorders. Women over the age of sixty are a high risk. In some cases, children develop thyroid disorders, more often in infancy.

Autoimmune Diseases: If you have any autoimmune disease like rheumatoid arthritis, multiple sclerosis, or others, you are at a high risk of developing thyroid disorders. Again, if any of your family members have autoimmune disease or glandular problems like goiter, you could develop thyroid disorders.

Hormonal Change: Women undergo various hormonal changes in a lifetime. Changes occur due to puberty, pregnancy, childbirth, perimenopause, and menopause. Post-partum and menopausal periods are the most vulnerable periods for thyroid problems to surface. Even otherwise, these periods of hormonal changes makes a woman susceptible to thyroid disorders.

Medications: Certain medications specifically those of high blood pressure, heart ailments, and psychiatric problems cause thyroid disorders.

Iodine Deficiency: Insufficient levels of iodine in diet could lead to thyroid disorders. However presently iodine is available in your diet and hence this deficiency does not hold great importance.

Previous Thyroid Problems: If you have had any thyroid related problems like goiter, or thyroid disorders, you stand a greater risk of developing it again. If you have undergone surgery to remove a part of thyroid or undergone therapy to resolve thyroid problems anytime in the past, you could develop thyroid problems again.

Medical Treatment: If you have undergone radiation therapy or treatments for any problems in brain and neck region, you could develop thyroid issues. Radiation rays often lead to thyroid gland problems.

Pregnant Women: If you have had thyroid problems sometime in the past, you could develop it again during pregnancy. Sometimes, it develops within the first year of childbirth.

Men with Hormonal Problems: Men with enlarged breasts or Gynecomastia or men with erectile dysfunction could develop thyroid disorders. Hormonal imbalances in body cause such diseases.

===\\\===\\\===\\\===\\\===\\\===\\\===

45. Is Thyroid Disease Curable?

Thyroid diseases are curable. Hyperthyroidism is over-activation of thyroid gland leading to excess hormones in blood. Hypothyroid is under-activation of thyroid gland leading to deficiency of hormones in blood. Other thyroid diseases include immune system malfunctions, cancers, nodules, and tumors.

Most thyroid diseases occur more commonly in women than in men. Although female hormone estrogen does play a role, other factors are also responsible for thyroid diseases. Irrespective of whichever thyroid disease affects you, you can be cured. There is increased awareness about thyroid gland.

Thyroid cancer is a curable cancer. This cancer spreads very slowly. I advise simple radiotherapy treatment to cure thyroid cancer. Often people with thyroid cancer die only due to other diseases.

===\\\===\\\===\\\===\\\===\\\===\\\===

46. Treating a Hypothyroidism Patient

If you have hypothyroidism, you will be on thyroid hormone replacement for your entire life. Medications in correct dosage ease your symptoms. Blood tests show T4 and TSH at normal levels and your overall health improves. There are different brands and varieties of hormone replacement drugs. Your doctor not only suggests specific brand and variety but also the correct dosage to bring back your thyroid hormones at acceptable levels.

Hypothyroid Drugs

Synthetic T4

Your body can easily convert T4 into T3. Although T3 is the more active form of thyroid hormone, T4 is more stable. T3 drugs are normally responsible for sudden highs and lows of thyroid hormone in blood.

Synthetic T4, Levothyroxine, is available under different brands. However, Synthroid is the most popular and prescribed brand. Other brands include Unithroid, Levoxyl, and Levothroid. All brands contain synthetic thyroxin. Levothyroxine is available in different color dosage. It is normally white in color and does not contain any dyes. Normal dosage is a single pill. Follow your doctor's advice and take pills as prescribed. Synthetic thyroxin has similar characteristics as actual T4 secreted in your body. T4 provides a steady supply of thyroid hormone to all body cells as it remains in your blood for a long time.

Treatment with T4 alone proves sufficient and successful for most people with hypothyroidism. Normally soon after starting with T4 pills, your TSH comes back to normal levels and you no longer suffer from hypothyroidism symptoms. If symptoms do not go away, I would suggest treatment with T3 also.

Synthetic T3

T3 is the more active form of thyroid hormone. Synthetic T3, Liothyronine, is available under brand name Cytomel. T3 remains in body for very less time. Hence, you need many doses in a day to reap the best benefits. If you need to undergo whole body scan, your hypothyroid symptoms should be lessened. Synthetic T3 is useful here.

Synthetic T3 as medication for hypothyroidism interrupts regulation of TSH levels. Further, if you take only T3, T4 levels will drop. Again, excessive T3 is harmful for heart. Nonetheless, T3 is essential to treat hypothyroidism even if synthetic T4 has been able to normalize TSH levels.

Use of T3 is extremely controversial. Some are of the view that hypothyroid people should take both T4 and T3. If free T3 levels in blood are low, synthetic T3 treatment could yield positive results. If you are on synthetic T4 and synthetic T3, you should maintain free T3 and free T4 at normal levels. This combination lowers TSH levels as T3 suppresses TSH.

Combination of Synthetic T4 and T3

This combination drug is liotrix available under brand name Thyrolar. Ratio of T3 to T4 in Thyrolar is 1 to 4. Ratio remains fixed in combination drug. However, if you take T3 or T4 separately, your doctor can adjust ratios to suit your requirements. Nonetheless, some do not find relief in this combination treatment. Often, there is no difference between T4 treatment alone and combination treatment.

Desiccated Thyroid Drugs

Armour is the most renowned brand of desiccated thyroid drugs. It was the only thyroid hormone drug available in early and middle twentieth century. Even after synthetic thyroid drugs entered the market, Armour remains a popular treatment option for hypothyroid people. Armour is much cheaper than synthetic thyroid hormone. Although Armour is the most popular brand, others include Nature-Throid, Westhroid, and Bio-Throid.

Hormones extracted from thyroid glands of pigs are used in making desiccated thyroid drugs. Since these contain natural hormones, such drugs are often more effective. Nonetheless, some doctors are skeptical of prescribing them. Since thyroid hormone is derived from pigs, hormone consistency could differ across different pigs and this discrepancy would be present in the drug. Such problems do not exist in synthetic drugs. However, Armour harps on same consistency in every pill.

If hypothyroid symptoms do not improve with either synthetic T4 alone or a combination of T4 and T3, I would suggest a combination of Armour with synthetic T4.

Important Points to Consider

◻ Your thyroid hormone replacement drug dosage should be in direct relation to your weight. If you weigh more, dosage should be high.

◻ Dosage of replacement drugs for elderly people and those with heart ailments should start with a low dose to allow body to adjust to the drug. Often, dosage for such people continues to be at low levels unless your doctor prescribes higher dosage to solve your hypothyroidism problems.

▫ Dosage also depends on the cause for your hypothyroidism. If your thyroid secretes small quantities of hormone, I would suggest a lower dose of synthetic thyroid drug. However, if your thyroid gland has been removed, you would need a high dosage of the drug.

▫ Take drugs consistently. If you miss a dose, take it as soon as you remember. If you take drugs containing T3, follow dosage of twice to thrice a day.

▫ Do not eat anything for an hour after taking your pill. This helps easy absorption of thyroid hormone.

===\\\===\\\===\\\===\\\===\\\===\\\===

47. Treating a Hyperthyroidism Patient

Hyperthyroidism requires immediate and effective treatment as untreated hyperthyroidism leads to bone loss and heart ailments. Different drugs suit different hyperthyroidism patients. Hence, consult your doctor about which hyperthyroidism drug would be most effective for your condition.

Hyperthyroidism Treatment Options

Your treatment depends on severity of your condition, type of hyperthyroidism you have, and your response to available treatments.

Treatment options include:

Radioactive Iodine (RAI)

This treatment destroys a part or whole of thyroid tissue that produces excess thyroid hormone. You should undergo a RAIU (Radioactive iodine ultrasound) scan before starting with RAI treatment. The scan confirms that you suffer from hyperthyroidism and not thyroiditis. RAIU uses a stronger radioactive isotope, iodine-131, instead of iodine-123. If you start with low levels of RAI, you should take Thyrogen. This synthetic TSH encourages thyroid cells to take RAI.

Before starting with RAI treatment, eat a low-iodine diet for few weeks. This prevents other sources of iodine from interfering with RAI. Normally, nuclear medicine division of a hospital administers RAI either in the form of a liquid or pill. RAI reaches overactive thyroid cells through the bloodstream. Soon it destroys diseased thyroid tissue.

RAI is excreted through saliva, urine, and sweat. Although radioactivity is substantially small, you should take specific precautionary steps so that radioactivity does not contaminate others.

Important Precautionary Measures

◻ Stay away from pregnant women and children. Try to maintain sufficient distance from other people also.
◻ Drink lots of water to flush away RAI from your system.
◻ Flush toilets twice or thrice after each use.
◻ Sleep alone.
◻ Keep your towels, clothes, and linens separately.
◻ Use separate utensils to cook for yourself.
◻ Wash utensils and vessels soon after use.
◻ Preferably use throw away plates and cups.
◻ Do not prepare food for others.
◻ If you have to travel by air soon after RAI treatment, carry a letter from your doctor detailing your recent therapy treatment. Even the smallest amount of radioactive element present in your body can trigger certain devices in plane.

Effectiveness of RAI Treatment

RAI treatment is extremely effective. Nonetheless, effectiveness is visible only after considerable time. You undergo regular blood tests to measure amount of thyroid hormone in your blood. Your symptoms fade away completely after few months.

Overall, RAI treatment is safe and effective. A complete dose of RAI treatment is effective for most people with hyperthyroidism. Some requires a second dose. In very rare instances, a third dose is necessary.

RAI treatment does not perpetuate thyroid cancer. High doses of RAI offer remedial solutions to cure your hyperthyroidism. However, it is common to turn hypothyroid after RAI treatment. Yet small doses of RAI does not offer full cure and you continue to suffer from hyperthyroidism symptoms. Nonetheless, thyroid levels return to normalcy in some people after RAI treatment. This stays for a year or two and thereafter you develop either hypothyroidism or hyperthyroidism.

Side Effects of RAI Treatment

Common side effects include:

□ Nausea
□ Dryness in the mouth
□ Vomiting
□ Pain or tenderness in the neck
□ Lower secretion of saliva

Some experience an increase in hyperthyroidism symptoms. Diseased cells destroyed by RAI treatment spill thyroid hormones into blood. This increases hormone levels in blood leading to an increase in hyperthyroidism symptoms. Elderly people are more prone to such problems. Existing heart ailments further compound symptoms. However, this is a temporary phase and you soon overcome such symptoms. Anti-thyroid drugs can relieve symptoms.

Essential Precautions of RAI Treatment

□ Pregnant women should not undergo RAI treatment.
□ Women should not conceive within a year of treatment.

▫ If you suffer from eye ailments, do not go for RAI treatment. However, if RAI is extremely essential, take steroids to reduce impact on eyes.

Anti-Thyroid Drugs

Anti-thyroid drugs or Thionamides block thyroid hormone production and make it difficult for thyroid gland to use iodine. These drugs take a long time to be effective. Methimazole, available under brand name Tapazole, is an anti-thyroid drug. These drugs stabilize thyroid hormones at normal levels within two years. Normal dosage is twice or thrice a day. Nonetheless, dosage should be adjusted so that thyroid function gradually becomes normal. Often serious side effects like nausea and skin rashes deter regular intake of medications. In some cases, hyperthyroidism returns when drugs are stopped.

Surgery

If RAI treatment or anti-thyroid drugs do not deliver desired results, you should undergo surgery to cure hyperthyroidism. Depending on the severity of hyperthyroidism, either a part or the whole thyroid gland has to be removed.

If a part of thyroid gland is removed, you do not need any thyroid hormone replacement for life. If your thyroid gland is removed completely, you are no longer hyperthyroid but could certainly develop hypothyroidism.

Surgery has serious side effects and risks. These include:

▫ Hoarseness of voice
▫ Damage to parathyroid gland and vocal cords
▫ Depression

- Muscular pain
- Numbness
- Low calcium levels
- Pain in neck

===\\\===\\\===\\\===\\\===\\\===\\\===

48. Treating a Thyroid Nodules Patient

Thyroid nodules could be small, large, cysts, indeterminate, benign, or cancerous. Treatment options are decided accordingly.

Treating Thyroid Nodules

Very Small Nodules
I do not suggest any treatment for such small thyroid nodules. They do not cause any problem and often remain undetected.

Large Nodules
Big nodules are problematic. You are unable to swallow your food. You are unable to breathe easily while lying down or sleeping. Surgical removal of nodule is necessary.

Indeterminate Nodules
Sometimes it is not possible to determine the exact nature of thyroid nodules. Surgical removal of such nodules is the best option. I suggest removing part of thyroid gland that contains these nodules. Once removed, tissue examination can determine if it is malignant or not. If malignant, I suggest removal of entire thyroid gland to prevent cancer from spreading further.

Cysts
Cysts are small nodules. Nonetheless, they grow very fast. They cause pain and discomfort as they contain fluid. I suggest aspiration to treat such cysts. Fluid from cysts is removed with a syringe. Often fluid accumulates again within cysts. Hence, I suggest injecting ethanol into cysts after fluid removal. Cysts walls then stick together and there is no space for fluid accumulation.

Non-Cancerous or Benign Nodules

Biopsy of nodule reveals if thyroid nodule is cancerous or non-cancerous. If it is benign, I would only advise regular thyroid function tests and intermittent physical examination. If nodule does not grow, you do not require any further treatment. If nodule grows, another biopsy will decide necessary treatment.

Toxic Adenomas

This causes hyperthyroidism. Adenomas suppress TSH functioning. A beta-blocker can reduce mild symptoms. Normally, these nodules are not completely cured with mild medications. They reoccur with greater tenacity. I suggest radioactive iodine in liquid form or as a capsule. Your gland absorbs the iodine and symptoms subside within two to three months. Thyroid hormone level falls and TSH level starts increasing, rather TSH starts functioning. However, radioactive iodine treatment does not suit everybody. If you are pregnant or have large adenomas, I would suggest surgery to remove a part or whole of thyroid gland. Subsequent medication would ensure nodule does not reoccur.

Hyperthyroidism

I suggest medications like Methimazole or Tapazole to reduce thyroid hormone levels. You should take medicines for a long period. Side effects include liver problems.

Thyroid Cancer

Surgical removal of affected thyroid tissue, Thyroidectomy, is the best option. This often damages nerves of vocal cord and parathyroid glands. These tiny glands control calcium levels in blood. After Thyroidectomy, you should continue with Levothyroxine for your entire life to provide and maintain thyroid hormone at normal levels.

Thyroid Hormone Suppression Therapy

This is effective at shrinking thyroid nodules. Nonetheless, this therapy should be implemented only after careful evaluation of thyroid disease and your general health.

===\\\===\\\===\\\===\\\===\\\===\\\===

49. Treating a Thyroiditis Patient

Treatment for thyroiditis is according to type of thyroiditis. It spreads over three phases:

1. Overactive phase
2. Underactive phase
3. Return to normalcy

Treatments

Hashimoto's Thyroiditis
I suggest immediate hormone replacement like thyroxin and non-steroidal anti-inflammatory medications to prevent gland from further swelling. I would also prescribe few beta-blockers to reduce heartbeat rate and tremors. Bed rest is necessary.

Thyrotoxicosis
This is a temporary phase when gland is not over-active and hence anti-thyroid medications are not necessary. Instead, I suggest beta-blockers to restrict tremors and palpitations. Medications should be tapered off as symptoms improve.

Thyroidal Pain
The most common symptom of serious sub acute thyroiditis is pain in thyroid gland. Anti-inflammatory medications like ibuprofen and aspirin provide relief. If pain is very severe, I advise steroid therapy with prednisone.

Hypothyroidism

If you suffer from simple symptoms of post-partum hypothyroidism or sub acute hypothyroidism, I would not suggest any treatment at all as these symptoms often die away by themselves. If you have serious symptoms, I advise thyroid hormone therapy. Treatment should continue for six to twelve months and thereafter tapered off slowly. If it is a large goiter, I advise Levothyroxine.

Surgery
I suggest surgery only in rare cases. Often, partial thyroid removal is the best solution in such cases.

Complementary and Alternative Therapies
There are several complementary and alternative therapies for treating a thyroiditis patient. Such therapies cannot be used as primary treatment options. Discuss with your doctor before starting on such therapies and medications as often they interfere with regular medications.

===\\\===\\\===\\\===\\\===\\\===\\\===

50. Treating a Thyroid Cancer Patient

Thyroid cancer treatment depends on type and stage of your thyroid cancer and your overall health. Few types of thyroid cancer in the elderly are very slow growing and have hardly any symptoms. I do not advise any treatment for such cancer. Almost all types of thyroid cancer can be treated. They are not fatal unless cancer has spread to almost all body parts.

Once you are diagnosed with thyroid cancer, you should detect its stage to plan your treatment. Cancer stage depends on size of tumor, spread of cancer, and your age. Normally cancer spreads less in the young and more in the elderly. Chances of survival are high when cancer spread is low. Nonetheless, thyroid cancer is less fatal than other forms of cancer and can be easily treated.

Treatments for Thyroid Cancer

Surgery

Surgeon makes an incision at the base of your neck. Operation extends for around two hours. Thereafter you should stay at hospital for three to seven days. Surgery could be:

Lobectomy: If cancerous nodule is small and restricted to just a single lobe, treatment involves removing the lobe alone.

Subtotal Thyroidectomy: If cancer has spread to both lobes, treatment involves removing almost the entire thyroid gland. Nonetheless, important nerves and some tissue around parathyroid glands are left behind to prevent any damage to parathyroid glands and nerves.

Total Thyroidectomy: However, if cancer has spread extensively, treatment involves removing the entire thyroid gland. This is the most common treatment for thyroid cancer. Enlarged lymph nodes from your neck are also removed and tested for cancer.

Surgery complications include:

□ Temporary or permanent hoarseness
□ Excessive bleeding
□ Vocal cord paralysis
□ Infection
□ Difficulty in breathing
□ Damage to parathyroid glands leading to low calcium levels and muscular spasms
□ Numbness or tingling

Thyroid Hormone Therapy

After surgery, I advise medications for thyroid hormones replacement like Levothyroxine or Levothroid, Synthroid, and others. Dosage should be appropriate enough to keep TSH at low levels and thyroid hormones at required levels. You should carry on with these medications all through your life.

Radioactive Iodine Treatment

Sometimes thyroid cancer spreads to other body parts or recurs after treatment. Sometimes microscopic areas of thyroid cancer are not removed during surgery. These are treated through radioactive iodine 131. This is in the form of a liquid or capsule. The iodine is absorbed by thyroid cancer cells. Hence, other body cells remain unharmed.

Before starting with this treatment, you should eat a diet low in iodine and discontinue thyroid hormone pills. This increases TSH levels, which are very essential for treatment to be effective. Low iodine levels in diet restrict any interference of ingested iodine with iodine in RAI.

The first dose of RAI, ablation dose, is usually given around six weeks after surgery. This removes any leftover thyroid tissue. Thereafter treatment plans depend on your medical condition. You might need to stay in the hospital for two or three days. In some cases, treatment is also possible as an outpatient.

Common side effects include:

▫ Dry mouth
▫ Nausea
▫ Dry eyes
▫ Pain across chest or neck if thyroid cancer cells have spread
▫ Change in sense of taste or smell

Radioactive iodine is excreted as urine soon after your treatment. During this time, you should follow certain restrictions:

▫ Avoid close contact with children and pregnant women
▫ Bathe daily
▫ Use private toilets
▫ Wash hands frequently
▫ Use disposable eating utensils
▫ Sleep alone
▫ Launder your linens separately
▫ Do not prepare food for others

External Radiation Therapy

If thyroid cancer has spread to your bones, external radiation therapy is beneficial. You lie on a table and a machine aims high-energy beams at precise points on your body for few minutes. This treatment spreads across five days each week, normally extending to six weeks.

Chemotherapy

This treatment is normally not used for thyroid cancer. However, if you do not respond to regular thyroid cancer treatments, chemotherapy becomes essential. Chemicals are infused through your vein. They travel very fast throughout your body and kill cancer cells. This treatment can at times damage nearby tissue. Side effects include skin damage and extensive fatigue.

===\\\===\\\===\\\===\\\===\\\===\\\===

51. Treating a Goiter Patient

Treatment for goiter depends on your symptoms, size of goiter, and the main cause behind goiter.

If your thyroid gland is functioning normally and your goiter is very small and does not cause any problems, I would not advise any treatment right now. It is better to wait and watch if goiter progresses any further.

Treatment Options for Goiter

Medications

Levothyroxine from Levothroid or Synthroid are very effective medications for hypothyroidism. These regulate thyroid-stimulating hormone of pituitary gland. TSH levels fall and goiter size reduces. If your goiter is due to hyperthyroidism, you may take medications to reduce hormone levels. This would also reduce goiter size. Aspirin or corticosteroid pills are best medications to treat gland inflammation.

Radioactive Iodine

An overactive thyroid gland causes goiter. Oral ingestion of radioactive iodine available in the form of a pill or capsule reaches your thyroid gland through your blood. It thereby reduces goiter size. Sometimes radioactive iodine medications lead to hypothyroidism. I would then suggest you remain on synthetic thyroid hormone Levothyroxine for life. This treatment best suits the elderly, as they are often unable to bear surgery.

Surgery

If you have a large goiter that causes problems in swallowing and breathing, surgical removal of the whole or a part of thyroid gland (total or partial Thyroidectomy) is necessary.

If your entire or major part of thyroid gland is surgically removed, you should start and continue with Levothyroxine for life.

Hashimoto's Thyroiditis

If goiter develops due to Hashimoto's thyroiditis, I would suggest a daily dosage of thyroid hormone supplement. Although this does not clear away goiter completely, it diminishes it in size.

Thyroid hormone treatment does not allow it to grow any further. Your thyroid hormones return to normal levels.

Biopsy

If there are many nodules in thyroid gland, I would suggest removing gland tissue from these nodules for a biopsy. This medical examination of thyroid gland tissue will clarify if the cells are malignant or benign. If malignant, it indicates thyroid cancer.

I would then suggest surgical removal of entire thyroid gland.

Toxic Multinodular Goiters

Sometimes there are many nodules in your enlarged thyroid gland. These nodules normally do not shrink away with anti-thyroid medications. Although RAI and surgery are the best treatment options, sometimes, you may not be able to withstand these treatments.

I would then suggest a first course of treatment with lithium or recombinant TSH. This enhances iodine intake and you are able to withstand RAI treatment.

Nontoxic Goiters

If your goiter does not contain any toxicity, there is no need for any treatment at all. Nonetheless, if goiter is very large and causes problems due to its size, surgical removal is the best option. RAI can shrink goiter size appreciably.

Annual monitoring is essential if you have been diagnosed with goiter.

===\\\===\\\===\\\===\\\===\\\===\\\===

52. Thyroid Medications - Myths and Facts

1. Myth: Once you start with thyroid medications, you have to stay put with them for life.

Fact: Once thyroid medications bring down your hormone levels to normal levels, you can gradually wean off medications. Most thyroid disorders like postpartum thyroiditis or thyroiditis due to immune system ailments occur temporarily. You require medications only to overcome these disorders and thereafter can quit medications completely.

2. Myth: Only older women develop thyroid problems.

Fact: It is true that older women over the age of fifty or sixty have a higher chance of developing thyroid disorders due to various hormonal changes. Nonetheless, even young women develop post-partum thyroiditis soon after childbirth. Women in the thirties are also vulnerable to thyroid disorders. Further, men could also develop thyroid disorders as they age.

3. Myth: Graves' disease or hyperthyroidism leads to bulging eyes.

Fact: Bulging eyes is one of the symptoms of Graves' disease. It is not mandatory for everyone diagnosed with Graves' disease to develop bulging eyes. Sometimes people with hypothyroidism also have bulging eyes. It is also true that people with eye disorders have bulging eyes although they have a perfectly normal thyroid gland.

4. Myth: TSH test is the only accurate way to diagnose a thyroid problem.

Fact: TSH is a diagnostic test to detect thyroid disorder. However, it cannot be accepted as the only tool to detect thyroid disorder. Often, thyroid symptoms present a clearer picture of the disorder than TSH test. In many cases, underactive thyroids display normal TSH levels. Hence, it is best to arrive at a diagnosis through coordinated study of existing symptoms, blood test, and physical examination rather than judging by TSH levels alone.

5. Myth: A lump or nodule in the thyroid means you have thyroid cancer.

Fact: Only around five percent of thyroid nodules are cancerous. Just a nodule or lump in your thyroid gland does not cause thyroid cancer.

6. Myth: Iodine deficiency is a medical problem.

Fact: Iodine deficiency is not any medical problem. Rather, it is a social problem. Your body gets iodine from your diet. Certain foods like cassava reduce iodine content in your body. Hence, people should be educated about iodine-rich foods and foods that reduce iodine in your body so that iodine intake is sufficient.

7. Myth: I cannot lose weight since I have hypothyroidism or I cannot gain weight since I have Hyperthyroidism.

Fact: Hypothyroidism and hyperthyroidism cause changes in your weight. However, blaming these thyroid disorders alone for your weight changes is not fair.

Often age plays an important role, as your metabolism rates falls and you are less physically active. These contribute to your weight gain. Again, not all hyperthyroid people lose weight. Instead, some gain weight.

===\\\===\\\===\\\===\\\===\\\===\\\===

Part-V: The Nutrition-Based Approach for Thyroid Management

53. Hashimoto's Disease is an Immune Disease, Not a Thyroid Disease

Hashimoto's thyroiditis is the first disease to be recognized as an autoimmune disease of thyroid gland. This endocrine gland produces various hormones that coordinate many activities of your body. Hashimoto's thyroiditis is same as chronic lymphocytic thyroiditis. It is the most common cause of hypothyroidism in the United States.

In Hashimoto's disease, your immune system attacks your thyroid gland. This inflames the gland and your thyroid is unable to produce required amount of hormones. It restricts growth in children and adolescents. An underactive thyroid leads to hypothyroidism. There is no clear medical evidence as to what causes your immune system to attack your thyroid gland. It could be due to bacteria, virus, or an inborn genetic disorder.

Who gets Hashimoto's Disease?

Although Hashimoto's disease can affect people of any age, women are seven times more prone to it than men. Again, it is extremely common among middle-aged women. Sometimes young teenage girls are also affected by this disorder. Nonetheless, you are at a greater risk of Hashimoto's disease if you or your family members have any autoimmune diseases like:

Rheumatoid Arthritis: This slowly erodes lining of joints all through your body.

Vitiligo: This destroys cells that are responsible for color of your skin.

Type 1 Diabetes: This increases blood sugar levels excessively.

Graves' Disease: This increases thyroid hormone production.

Addison's Disease: This is a disease of adrenal glands. These glands produce hormones to regulate your blood pressure and maintain appropriate salt and water balance in body. These hormones also control your stress levels.

Lupus: This autoimmune disease affects many body parts like skin, joints, blood vessels, and other major organs.

Pernicious Anemia: This leads to severe anemic condition as this disease prevents your body from absorbing vitamin B12. Hence, your body is unable to create sufficient and healthy red blood cells.

Diagnosis of Hashimoto's Disease

Diagnosis of Hashimoto's disease is normally through an antibody test. It detects presence of antibodies against a body enzyme, thyroid peroxidase. This thyroid gland enzyme is responsible for production of thyroid hormones.

What if Hashimoto's disease is left untreated?

Untreated Hashimoto's disease slowly progresses into hypothyroidism as your thyroid gland produces fewer hormones. You exhibit various symptoms like:

□ Excessive tiredness
□ Lethargy
□ Constipation

▫ Puffy face
▫ Increased intolerance to cold
▫ Excessive or prolonged menstrual bleeding
▫ Dry skin
▫ Hoarse voice
▫ Excessive weight gain
▫ Depression

Prolonged and untreated Hashimoto's disease causes serious disorders like high cholesterol, lymphoma of thyroid gland, miscarriage, infertility, giving birth to baby with birth defects, forgetfulness, and others. In extreme cases, it could lead to a condition called myxedema. This causes seizures, heart failure, coma, and eventual death.

===\\\===\\\===\\\===\\\===\\\===\\\===

54. Connection between Your Blood Sugar Level and Thyroid Health

Hypoglycemia is a condition where blood sugar levels are low. Hyperglycemia is a condition where blood sugar levels are high. Changes in body blood sugar levels affect secretion of hormones in thyroid gland. This eventually leads to thyroid disorders.

What is Hypoglycemia?

Hypoglycemia is a condition where your blood sugar levels fall down considerably. Blood sugar levels are detected through blood tests. Fasting blood glucose measures your blood sugar before eating or drinking anything in the morning. 100 mg/dL is considered normal fasting blood glucose. Post-prandial blood glucose measures your blood sugar two hours after a meal. 120 mg/dL is considered normal post-prandial blood glucose.

Common hypoglycemia symptoms include:

□ constant feeling of hunger
□ headaches
□ rapid heartbeat
□ double vision
□ convulsions

Sometimes, blood tests reveal normal levels but you exhibit all symptoms of hypoglycemia.

Causes behind Hypoglycemia

1. Your diet is the main cause behind hypoglycemia. If you eat refined foods and sugars often, it pushes insulin levels. This in turn is responsible for increasing blood sugar levels. Sensing high blood sugar levels, adrenal glands secrete cortisol to push down sugar levels in your blood. Eating such foods regularly pressurizes functioning of pancreas and adrenal glands. Eventually you become hypoglycemic.

2. Skipping meals creates a similar situation and leads to hypoglycemia.

3. Chromium is an important mineral essential for normal insulin functioning. It also helps in the breaking down of carbohydrates, fats, and protein. If you are deficient in chromium, breakdown of fats, carbohydrates, and protein is affected. Further, insulin utilization is also affected. This leads to hypoglycemia.

4. Deficiency of thyroid hormone as prevalent in those with Hashimoto's Thyroiditis and hypothyroidism also leads to hypoglycemia. Thyroid hormone stimulates glucose-genesis or absorption of glucose through proper synthesis.

5. Weak adrenal glands also cause hypoglycemia. These glands produce cortisol and epinephrine. They also affect secretion of thyroid hormones. Hence, weak adrenal glands affect secretion of all these hormones. Eventually this led to hypoglycemia.

6. Thyroid hormone affects liver functioning. Poor secretion of thyroid hormones disrupts liver functioning. Further, excess glucose in body is stored in the liver. Malfunctioning of liver affects storage of glucose. Such a liver often leads to hypoglycemia.

What is Hyperglycemia?

Hyperglycemia is a condition where your blood sugar levels shoot up considerably. Your blood sugar levels should be below 120 mg/dL two hours after a meal to maintain normal hyperglycemic levels.

Excessive intake of carbohydrates stimulates pancreas to secrete more insulin to help remove glucose from blood and store them in cells to convert them into energy. However, prolonged intake of excessive carbohydrates hampers normal functioning of pancreas and insulin. Body cells are unable to utilize insulin effectively. This increases blood sugar levels leading to hyperglycemia.

Pancreas tries to normalize situation by producing excess insulin. Eventually this leads to insulin resistance. Insulin resistance leads to frequent ups and downs in insulin levels in body. This affects your thyroid gland. The effect is higher if you have an autoimmune disease. All together disrupt thyroid gland functioning and production of thyroid hormones.

Interconnection between Hypoglycemia, Hyperglycemia, and Thyroid Health

Hyperglycemia and hypoglycemia are together referred to as dysglycemia. Dysglycemia is responsible for various far-reaching effects like:

□ Inflammation and weakening of gut
□ Hormonal level imbalance
□ Weakening of lungs and brain
□ Adrenal gland malfunctioning
□ Disrupting normal detoxification process
□ Impairing normal metabolism

All together, these affect functioning of thyroid gland. Hence, if you suffer from dysglycemia, medications and treatment for thyroid gland do not deliver desired results.

Hypothyroidism left untreated increases cholesterol levels in blood. Medications can bring down cholesterol levels in blood. Yet, genetic factors and improper or irregular diet habits could prevent effective control of cholesterol. If you have type I diabetes, your thyroid hormone secretion will be low leading to hypothyroidism. Autoimmune diseases further hamper functioning of pancreas and thyroid gland. Again, hyperthyroidism pushes blood sugar levels excessively due to high metabolism rate. You need more insulin to keep blood sugar at normal levels. At the same time, insulin levels should be low to check hyperthyroidism.

An effective coordination of hypothyroidism, hyperthyroidism, and blood sugar is essential to manage your thyroid health.

===\\\===\\\===\\\===\\\===\\\===\\\===

55. Why is Health of Your Gut Vital to a Healthy Thyroid?

Your gut plays an important role in not only your overall health but also your thyroid function. Around twenty percent of T4 is converted into T3 in your gut or intestines. Nonetheless, this is possible only if you have a healthy gut. If your gut is bloated and constipated, thyroid functions are hampered leading to thyroid disorders. It is common for people with thyroid disorders to have digestive problems. Leaky gut does not necessarily display gut symptoms. Often, autoimmune diseases like Hashimoto's thyroiditis, psoriasis, autism spectrum disorder, joint pains, or rheumatoid arthritis are symptoms of a leaky gut.

Gut Functioning and Your Health

1. It takes around twelve to twenty-four hours for food to pass from your mouth and to be excreted out. If it takes more than twenty-four hours, nutrient absorption is low. You have many food intolerances. You suffer from bacterial infections of gut. If it takes less than eighteen hours, your gut is unable to absorb all nutrients. Either way, you are not able to get the best of what you eat.

2. If you have a leaky gut, it is harmful to your thyroid. Drugs, sugary food, antibiotics, alcohol, and stress are few factors that start a leaky gut. Your gut or the digestive tract has numerous cells. When your gut swells, they dislodge from each other. Space between cells increases and small microscopic particles or proteins leak out from the tract into your bloodstream. These particles are not fully processed. This causes a leaky gut. The leaked out proteins move around freely and

settle within all types of body tissues. Thyroid gland is extremely susceptible to these proteins as it is floating in blood and thyroid hormones are circulated within your body through blood. Few proteins also settle within thyroid gland tissue. Since these proteins are foreign substances, your immune system attacks them. This leads to autoimmune disorders. These processes damage your thyroid gland. It functions slowly or sometimes malfunctions.

3. Gut has many probiotic good bacteria. Include more probiotic foods in your diet to improve health of your gut and thereby have a healthy thyroid gland. Your gut houses ten times more good bacteria than all the cells in your body. These bacteria are responsible for varied functions like protection from infection, normal gastrointestinal function, and effective metabolism. Absence of healthy gut bacteria is responsible for various diseases like inflammatory bowel disease, Hashimoto's thyroiditis, depression, type 1 diabetes, autism, and many others.

4. If you have a troublesome gut, avoid specific foods like eggs, dairy products, corn, gluten, yeast, and similar others. These foods cause gut allergies often leading to exaggerated immune responses like autoimmune disorders, blood sugar instability, weight gain, and associated thyroid problems.

Foods that Cause Gut Problems and Affect Thyroid Health

1. High glycemic fruits like mango, watermelon, bananas, canned fruits, raisins, dried fruits, and pineapple.

2. Grains like corn, barley, millet, rye, oats, buckwheat, quinoa, rice, wheat, and wheat germ.

3. Sugars like corn syrup, candy, fructose, chocolate, honey, high fructose corn syrup, molasses, and maple syrup.

4. Nuts and seeds like peanuts, almonds, sunflower seeds, and sesame seeds.

5. Dairy products like creams, butter, cheese, mayonnaise, yogurt, and eggs.

6. Soy as present in soy protein, soymilk, soy sauce, and tofu.

7. Beans and legumes like including lentils, black beans, peas, and soybeans.

8. Certain vegetables like peppers, tomatoes, eggplant, potatoes, paprika, and others.

Health Problems Related to Gut and Thyroid Gland

Your gut and thyroid gland are interrelated through their respective functions. Defect in any one leads to serious problems in the other. Hence, a healthy gut is essential for a healthy thyroid. Some of them include:

1. Hypothyroidism is often the cause behind poor gallbladder function. Gallbladder secretes bile. This is a digestive liquid that helps break down fats. It is also responsible for absorption of minerals into the gastrointestinal tract. Hypothyroidism leads to stones in gallbladder. Improper functioning of gallbladder affects your liver. Body detoxification is incomplete. T4 cannot be easily converted into T3 and excess estrogen is not eliminated. This affects thyroid hormone production leading to hypothyroidism.

2. Hypothyroidism causes hypochlorhydria. Acid levels in stomach are very low and food is not completely digested. Instead, you throw up.

This is extremely acidic for your esophagus and hence you suffer heartburn in your throat.

===\\\===\\\===\\\===\\\===\\\===\\\===

56. How Your Thyroid Health Depends on Adrenal Health

Your body has two adrenal glands, each of the size of a walnut. These glands produce cortisol and DHEA. They also help in producing hormones like testosterone, estrogen, progesterone, and others. Stress is the most important debilitating factor of adrenal glands. Regular and chronic stress slowly erodes away the strength and abilities of adrenal glands. This in turn affects functioning of your thyroid gland. Managing stress is an effective way to manage health of your adrenal and thyroid glands.

Functional Relationship between Adrenal and Thyroid Glands

Adrenal and thyroid are endocrine glands producing different body hormones. These glands function as sensors. There are numerous functions going on in your body constantly. These glands increase or decrease hormone secretion according to needs of your body and instructions as perceived from the brain and nervous system. Normally, they secrete only as much hormones as is necessary.

Both adrenal and thyroid glands function in loops relating to pituitary gland and hypothalamus in the brain. Hormones produced along these axes interact. Hence, if any one loop is overactive or underactive, hormones deregulate on the other loop. An over-production or underproduction of any hormone affects function of the other gland. Often, your thyroid levels are normal according to pathological reports, yet you display thyroid disorder symptoms. This is due to malfunctioning of adrenal gland affecting the loop.

How Stress Affects Functioning of Adrenal and Thyroid Glands

Stress is cited as the main cause for hyperthyroidism as in Graves' disease. This autoimmune disorder prompts thyroid gland to produce hormones in excess. Nonetheless, stress is often the cause behind hypothyroidism or poor production of thyroid hormone as stress slows down functioning of thyroid gland.

Stress of any kind, physical or mental, prompts your brain to release corticotrophin-releasing hormone or CRH. This hormone instructs pituitary gland to produce cortisol to combat stress. However, cortisol and CRH restrict functioning of thyroid gland and conversion of T4 into T3. This leads to a fall in circulation of T3 hormones in blood. T3 hormones are essential for almost every activity in body cells. Hence, poor T3 levels cause various symptoms like:

□ Fatigue
□ Weight gain
□ Cold intolerance
□ Memory loss
□ Depression
□ Hair loss
□ Infertility

Prolonged stress is often the main cause behind major health problems. Stress inhibits thyroid functions and often symptoms present much later.

Tips to Combat Stress for Healthy Adrenal and Thyroid Glands

1. Eat healthy foods like whole grain cereals, fruits, vegetables, and high-protein snacks. Restrict consumption of sugar and sugary foods, refined foods, and caffeine.

2. You should never skip breakfast and stick to specified timings of food intake. Restrict late and heavy dinners; instead have a heavy breakfast, and a moderately heavy lunch. Include high-protein snacks in between mealtimes.

3. Reduce stress levels by adopting simple techniques like massaging, yoga, meditation, walking, and breathing exercises. Maintain a schedule of these activities and adhere to them regularly. However, restrict everything within limits as overexertion of physical exercises prompts adrenal gland to produce more cortisol.

4. Sleep well and stick to a regular schedule of around eight hours of sleep. Relax with a book before going to bed. Allow short naps in between during daytime. This helps adrenal gland regulate hormone secretion and it remains competent enough to handle sudden emergencies without breaking down.

5. Provide your body with sufficient vitamins and minerals like iodine, vitamins A, B, C, and E, and selenium. All help in maintaining thyroid hormone production at normal levels. B vitamins and other vitamins like C and E are actively involved in producing stress hormones. Trace minerals like manganese, zinc, and iodine, selenium, and calcium lower stress levels in body and keep you calm. Magnesium provides essential energy to body cells and adrenal glands. All together help reduce any imbalance in adrenal gland secretion and maintain optimum cortisol production.

6. It is best to do strenuous exercises early in the morning or little later. Exercises increase cortisol production and this excess production is utilized over the day so that it does not upset your sleep pattern at night.

===\\\===\\\===\\\===\\\===\\\===\\\===

57. How Good Thyroid Nutrition Affects the Way You Feel

Nutrition is an essential part of your existence. It helps you handle diseases and combat them. Stick to a balanced diet including fats, proteins, carbohydrates, vitamins, and minerals. Further, eat food regularly. Follow a daily routine and eat food at almost the same time each day. Stay away from junk food. Following such a pattern of food habits will help you overcome thyroid diseases.

Carbohydrates

Carbohydrates are the most important source of energy. Simple carbohydrates are present in milk, low-fat dairy products, fruits, and vegetables in their natural form. These offer instant energy as they break down easily.

Complex carbohydrates are contained in grains, legumes, oats, and certain vegetables like beans, potatoes, and lentils. These contain starches that are broken down into simple sugars by your body. This process takes time and hence these carbohydrates provide energy over few hours.

Fibrous foods cannot be converted into simple sugars, as they cannot be digested in the stomach. Your body does not take any energy from fibrous foods; instead, it is excreted. Rather fibrous foods help alleviate problems of digestive disorders.

For best results, include fruits and vegetables in your daily diet and limit complex carbohydrates to reduce weight gain and lower cholesterol levels. Restrict intake of refined sugars as present in cookies, ice-cream, cakes, sweetened sugars, potato chips, and juices. Restrict consumption of vegetables and fruits like cabbage, broccoli, peaches, cauliflower, strawberries, spinach, radishes, and turnips.

Protein

Your body extracts energy from protein foods if it does not get enough energy from carbohydrates or fats. Proteins provide amino acids that are essential to build and repair body tissues. It ensures healthy muscle and tissues if you combine it with sufficient strength training.

Protein-rich foods include eggs, meat, seeds, legumes, nuts, soybeans, and tofu. Protein foods make you feel full and consequently you do not overeat. Often with thyroid disorders, you always feel hungry and crave for food. Protein foods help satiate your hunger better. It curbs your urge to eat and restricts weight gain. Excess protein remains stored as fat in your body.

Fats

Fats are essential for normal growth and functioning of brain and nervous tissue. Fats are concentrated forms of energy and provide almost double the amount of energy provided by carbohydrates or proteins.

Fats could be monounsaturated, unsaturated, saturated, and trans-fatty acids. Monounsaturated are the healthiest of all fats as available in olive oil and avocados. Polyunsaturated fats are found in vegetable oils like sunflower, safflower, and corn. They are less healthy than monounsaturated. Omega-3 fatty acids found in fish are a healthy form of polyunsaturated fat.

Saturated fats as available in wholesome dairy foods, meat, butter, coconut, and palm oils are not healthy. They clog your arteries. Trans-Fatty Acids are produced when oils are hydrogenated to solidify them at room temperature. These are present in processed foods like potato chips, breakfast cereals, crackers, frozen pancakes, and cookies.

Fats should be eaten in moderation to avoid weight gain. Further, avoid unhealthy fats as they lead to various diseases like heart ailments, cancer, and diabetes, to name a few.

Soy

Soy is termed as a plant estrogen. Soy is found in tempeh, tofu, soymilk, and soy sauce. Soy helps combat bone loss, hot flashes in menopausal women. It lowers cholesterol levels and fights against breast cancer. However, there are no clinical evidences to prove its effectiveness.

If you have hypothyroidism, excess soy could increase TSH levels leading to menstrual irregularities and goiter. It also restricts working of thyroid medications.

Vitamins and Minerals

Vitamins and minerals do not supply energy. However, they help in easy assimilation of energy from the foods you eat. Specific minerals help combat thyroid disorders. These include:

Iodine: This mineral is predominantly found in seafood, spinach, milk, eggs, and meat. You receive most of your iodine from iodized salt. If you do not have any thyroid problems, you can include lots of iodine in your diet. If you have hypothyroidism, excess iodine would restrict hormone production. If you have hyperthyroidism, excess iodine would worsen your symptoms further. If you are on a low-iodine diet, you would develop hypothyroidism. If you suffer from any chronic ailment, iodine absorption could be restricted. Regular thyroid tests help detect iodine levels in your body. If you have hypothyroidism, restrict red food dyes, shellfish, dairy products, multivitamins, and metabolic boosters.

Calcium: This mineral builds up your bones and helps muscles to contract. It also helps in clotting of blood. If calcium intake is less, your body uses calcium as available in your bones. This thins down your bones. Calcium is available from yogurt, low-fat milk, cheese, leafy green vegetables, orange juice, and canned fish with edible bones. If you have hyperthyroidism, excess thyroid hormones thin down your bones. Hence, you require additional calcium supplements. Restrict alcohol consumption as it reduces bone density. Further, alcohol consumption disturbs your coordination and balance raising risk of falls and fractures.

Selenium: This trace mineral exists naturally in soil. Selenium is found in seeds, nuts, and grains grown in such soil. It is also available in eggs, chicken, brown rice, walnuts, whole-wheat bread, and seafood. Selenium supplements improve autoimmune thyroiditis. It helps convert T4 to T3. Deficiency leads to hypothyroidism.

Iron: This mineral produces healthy red blood cells in your body and forms an essential part of hemoglobin. Iron also helps in converting T4 to T3. Deficiency causes anemia leading to fatigue, tiredness, and goiter. If you are on thyroid hormone medication, keep a gap of at least four hours before taking iron supplements.

===\\\===\\\===\\\===\\\===\\\===\\\===

Part-VI: Natural Remedies and Alternative Therapies for Thyroid Conditions

58. Neurological Treatments for Thyroid Based on Specific Neurological Testing

Normal brain functioning is of prime importance to thyroid health. A series of stimulating activities take place in your brain through the extensive network of nuclei. Hypothalamus in brain links your nervous system to endocrine system through pituitary gland. Hypothalamus sends TRH or thyroid releasing hormone to pituitary gland. Thereupon pituitary gland releases TSH or thyroid stimulating hormone to thyroid gland. TSH then stimulates TPO or thyroid peroxidase to create T4 and T3 hormones using iodine. Serotonin and dopamine are the important neurotransmitters of brain controlling these activities. Deficiency in any one of them impedes easy conversion of T4 to T3.

Neurological Treatments Based on Specific Neurological Testing

Oxygen therapy and brain-based therapy are important neurological treatments based on specific neurological testing.

Oxygen Therapy

Brain cannot store energy and requires a steady flow of oxygen and nutrients to maintain normal functions. Lack of sufficient oxygen reduces your memory, alertness, and judgment.

What is Oxygen Therapy?

Oxygen therapy is administration of oxygen to increase supply of oxygen to lungs so that body tissues receive adequate supply of oxygen to carry out normal activities. Oxygen is essential for cell metabolism and regular physiological functions. Oxygen fuels your brain and nervous system. This requires proper activation to improve brain functioning. If brain does not function normally, thyroid functions are affected. Oxygen therapy uses exercise with oxygen to activate your brain.

Cerebellum located in the backside of your brain controls spinal musculature, body balance, and overall coordinated movement of body muscles and tissues. Poor supply of oxygen disrupts this functioning. Muscles contract, disc loses fluid and degenerates, and vertebra lock up. Oxygen therapy corrects imbalance in oxygen supply and boosts systematic functioning of cerebellum.

Every cell in your body requires oxygen to live and carry out activities. Lungs transport oxygen to all body cells through airways. If there is any narrowing of airways or mucus, oxygen transportation is hampered. Your brain requires at least twenty percent of body's oxygen supply.

Exercise with Oxygen Therapy

This basic ability of your body to transfer oxygen from lungs to cells decides your health. Any damage to this transfer mechanism has far-reaching effects. Age also plays a role in debilitating this mechanism. Oxygen therapy restores this essential mechanism effectively to restore normal functioning and working of all body organs.

Oxygen therapy increases air circulation within your body. You breathe in high levels of oxygen while exercising. Arterial pressure increases. Exercise stimulates circulation. Oxygen flows through capillaries with greater pressure. This helps transfer mechanism to resume smooth functioning.

Tests to Determine Oxygen Therapy Requirements

Your oxygen level is measured as a percentage of oxygen in your blood. This is oxygen saturation. If this falls below ninety percent, you require oxygen therapy. There are two tests to determine oxygen saturation levels:

1. Oximetry: This involves a very easy and simple technique to determine your oxygen requirements. A small clip placed on your toe, finger, or earlobe determines your oxygen requirements.

2. Arterial Blood Gas Test: Blood is drawn from an artery in your wrist. Oxygen and carbon dioxide levels are measured. This indicates how your lungs are working. Although this test is more complex than oximetry, it provides more information.

The amount of oxygen you need is the flow rate and this differs during sleep, activity, and rest. Depending on test results, I suggest how much oxygen you need and how and when to use it.

Oxygen Systems

There are three oxygen systems, each with their own advantages and disadvantages. Choose a system that satisfies your requirements and fits within your lifestyle.

1. Compressed Gas Systems: These are in steel or aluminum cylinder tanks of varied sizes. They are easily available. Although smaller sizes are easily portable, this system proves little bulky.

2. Concentrators: You just plug into an electrical outlet and take oxygen from room air. This system is very convenient to use and can be transported anywhere. However, it is little noisy.

3. Liquid Systems: This system consists of two parts- a portable unit with a small lightweight tank and a large stationary container. You refill portable unit from the stationary unit and carry it along. Oxygen Supply Company refills stationary unit at periodic intervals.

Receiving Oxygen from Oxygen System

There are different methods to receive oxygen therapy. These include:

Trans-tracheal Oxygen Catheter: This is the best option if you require oxygen continuously for a long time and at a high flow rate. A thin tube placed in your neck delivers oxygen directly into your trachea or windpipe.

Cannula: This is a small plastic tube placed under your nostrils to deliver oxygen, similar to a facemask.

Hyperbaric Oxygen Therapy: This is very effective to treat common hypothyroid symptoms of poor concentration and brain fogginess. Poor metabolism rate and lack of quality oxygen to brain causes such symptoms. You would require a series of oxygen therapy sessions spread over a fortnight or more to improve hypothyroid symptoms and your overall health. This therapy is a costly option.

Brain-Based Therapy (BBT)

Brain Based Therapy or BBT is a healing technique based on natural factors used to restore brain functions for optimum coordination between different parts of brain and other organs of your body.

During normal functioning of brain, cerebellum sends messages to right and left hemispheres of brain. This is transmitted to the brainstem consisting of mesencephalon, pons, and medulla. This is 'Brain Loop'. If cerebellum does not receive sufficient inputs through nerves, it cannot send further inputs to brain stem. As a result, brain loop malfunctions. This causes symptoms like attention deficit disorder, fibromyalgia, poor concentration levels, depression, and others.

Further, cerebellum is responsible for controlling your balance, spinal postural muscles, and maintaining body and eye movements. An inactive cerebellum leads to spasms and imbalances in spinal movements. Individual vertebrae lock and free movement is restricted. This leads to arthritis, spinal degeneration, chronic back and neck pain, dizziness and balance disorders, and disc dislodgements.

A complete investigative BBT neurological examination and analysis detects which part of your brain is not functioning properly. Treatment is given accordingly to stimulate brain functioning. Traditional chiropractic instruments and adjustments are used to stimulate brain effectively. Other stimulation techniques used include auditory, visual, olfactory, eye movements, heat, and eye exercises.

Different Brain Based Therapies

There are different brain based therapies. Depending on your requirements, I would suggest any one or a combination of all these therapies for best results. Therapies include:

Laser Therapy: A laser is used to heal body tissues. This checks irregularities and brain functions return to normalcy.

Vibration Therapy: Vibration tactics help stimulate brain functions specifically those at back part of brain or cerebellum. Sometimes, a combination of visual, auditory, olfactory, and caloric stimulation revs up your brain and cerebellum. This improves functioning of spinal muscles.

Non-surgical Spinal Decompression (NSSD): This creates a negative disc pressure to remove pressure off the nerve. This helps muscles around spinal cord to stretch and function normally.

Interactive Metronome (IM): This is a computer-based program that uses auditory, visual, and motor stimulation to improve brain functions.

Brain functions through sympathetic and parasympathetic nervous systems. Sympathetic nervous system functions on 'fight or flight stress' response. Simple physical and emotional disturbances trigger this system. This works as a short-term response only. However, frequent activation of this system through stress, tension, exertion, and other factors weaken it. Characteristic symptoms include hypertension, palpitations, high cholesterol, high blood sugar, insomnia, anxiety, nervousness, headaches, concentration problems, and many others.

Parasympathetic nervous system helps relax and rejuvenate brain and body. When sympathetic nervous system is stressed, parasympathetic nervous system takes over and shifts body to a meditative state. Brain waves shift from beta to alpha and finally to deeply relaxed theta waves. This heals body hormones, activates them, and initiates thorough healing of body and mind.

Brain Therapy

Brain Wave Entrainment Therapy: This involves use of an audiovisual device. Every body part vibrates to its own waves of rhythm and frequencies like Beta, Alpha, Theta, and Delta. This device uses light flashes and pulse tones to improve symptoms of lack of sleep, concentration problems, mood swings, and poor relaxation. This therapy is individualistic and monitored according to your medical history and diagnosis.

Cranial-Electro Stimulation (CES): This simulative therapy reduces anxiety and improves sleep. CES device sends tiny impulses through a stimulation cable attached to earlobe to increase serotonin and endorphins. This calms your mind, improves sleep patterns, and reduces anxiety.

I also suggest various simple brain exercises according to individual patients to strengthen specific brain areas that are weak or not functioning well.

===\\\===\\\===\\\===\\\===\\\===\\\===

59. Metabolic Treatments for Thyroid Based on Specific Lab Panels

Metabolic treatments for thyroid disorders based on specific lab panels include:

Complete Thyroid Panel
Complete Thyroid Panel consists of TSH, Total T4, Free T4, Total T3, Free T3, antibodies, and FT index. If either the free hormones or any one of them is below the middle of lab range, it is a thyroid disorder irrespective of TSH value. Sometimes free Ts are well within mid-range and TSH could be little above 2 but below the upper limit while anti-thyroid antibodies and symptoms are present, I would advise starting thyroid treatment as antibodies indicate Hashimoto's disease and it will progress further. Normal ranges are:

◻ T4 Total: normal is 4.5-12.5
◻ TSH: normal is .3-3 (below is hyperthyroid and above is Hypothyroid)
◻ Free T4: normal is .58-1.64
◻ T3 Free: normal is 2.3-4.2
◻ Thyroid Peroxidase (Antibodies) normal is >35

Complete and Comprehensive Metabolic Panel or CMP
This blood test measures your electrolyte and fluid balance, sugar or glucose level, kidney and liver functions. It also measures blood levels of potassium, sodium, calcium, carbon dioxide, chloride, blood urea nitrogen, protein, creatinine, albumin, bilirubin, and liver enzymes. You should not eat or drink ten to twelve hours before you go for this blood test. This test detects medical conditions like diabetes, high blood pressure, and thyroid problems.

Lipid Panel

Lipids in your blood are normally stored in tissues. They help in normal body functions. Lipid Panel blood test measures lipids-fats like triglycerides, cholesterol, high-density lipoprotein or HDL (good cholesterol), low-density lipoprotein or LDL (bad cholesterol) and fatty substances used as a source of energy by your body. This test also measures ratio of total cholesterol to HDL, ratio of LDL to HDL, and very-low density lipoprotein or VLDL cholesterol level. You should not eat ten to twelve hours before you go for this blood test. You may drink water but do not drink any other liquid.

Complete Blood Count (CBC) with Differential

This blood test is a very common test. It records levels of white blood cells, red blood cells, platelet levels, hemoglobin, and hematocrit with differentials. Blood is collected in a test tube containing additive EDTA to prevent clotting. It provides complete and specific information about size, shape, and number of cells. This test is an important indicator of major ailments like anemia, and other blood conditions. However, lab ranges are extremely broad. Test results should be studied in perspective.

Sensitivity Testing

Gluten sensitivity refers to sensitivity to food groups like cereals, milk, eggs, yeast, and/or soy. Such sensitivity causes inflammation in brain and other body parts leading to frequent loose bowel movements, indigestion, constipation, fatigue, vomiting, and mouth ulcers or sores. A positive test shows an increased probability of immune system response. Celiac blood tests that detect gluten sensitivity indicate AGA-IgA and AGG-IgG or anti-gliadin antibodies. High levels indicate possibility of autoimmune disorders like autoimmune thyroid, type 1 diabetes, autoimmune hepatitis, and inflammatory bowel diseases.

Adrenal Stress Index or ASI

Adrenal glands are stress glands. Inactive or failing adrenal glands are due to chronic thyroid conditions. This test requires you to give four different saliva samples at different times during a single day. These tests detect your stress levels, problems of insomnia, and thyroid by measuring cortisol levels in your body. Additional tests evaluate glycemic control with the help of multiple salivary insulin measurements. Common symptoms of adrenal gland disorders include sleep disturbances, feeling of exhaustion, and sugar cravings. Test results combined with characteristic symptoms indicate adrenal gland disorders.

Autoimmune Disorders

Autoimmune disorder is when your immune system attacks and destroys healthy tissues of your body. A thyroid problem like Hashimoto's thyroiditis is an autoimmune disorder. Tests to detect autoimmune disorders include Autoantibody test, Antinuclear antibody test, CBC, Erythrocyte sedimentation rate (ESR), and C-reactive protein (CRP). Further tests required include detecting which part of your immune system is not functioning. This is possible through Lymphocyte subpopulation, Natural killer cell activity, and TH1/TH2 Cytokine panels. These tests deliver an in-depth insight into your actual condition. These coupled with physical examination can detect your medical condition.

Intestinal Permeability

This test determines if you suffer from leaky gut syndrome or LGS. This is a condition of damaged or changed bowel lining due to toxins, antibiotics, parasites, poor diet, or infection. This condition makes your vulnerable to increased permeability of gut wall by microbes, toxins, microbes, undigested food, and waste. Some of these affect your health directly while some propagate an immune reaction. Leaky gut syndrome can be tested through mannitol and lactulose test. If your intestinal linings are healthy, mannitol is easily absorbed. Lactulose is absorbed slightly since it is a larger molecule. You drink a solution containing both mannitol and lactulose. Urine is collected after six hours. It reflects how much was absorbed. High levels of mannitol and low levels of lactulose is a healthy indication. It is a leaky gut condition if high levels of both are found in urine. Low levels of both indicate poor absorption of all nutrients.

Helicobacter Pylori Test

Helicobacter Pylori is a bacterium that causes ulcers. This test determines problems related to gut functions. Often, thyroid disorders are due to poor gut health. H. pylori infections do not have any symptoms. Rather, symptoms are more of peptic ulcer disease or gastritis. Blood tests can detect presence of H. pylori antibodies. An endoscopic test of stomach lining detects infection and presence of H. pylori bacteria. Breath test detects carbon broken down by H. pylori after you drink specific solution. This test takes lot of time but does not provide any details of infection. Stool tests detect presence of H. pylori proteins in stool.

Hormone Panels

Testing these panels discloses hormone levels. Decreased hormone levels have various symptoms like mental fogginess, fatigue, depression, mood swings, weight gain, decreased physical stamina, and hot flashes. Regular assessment of hormone levels is very important and essential for women to maintain healthy hormonal balance. Hormonal status and endocrine function can be tested through the eight hormone panel of estradiol, progesterone, testosterone, DHEA and four cortisols. Hormonal imbalance has various symptoms like fatigue, irregular or severe periods, hot flashes, depression, night sweats, insomnia, and many others. A comprehensive hormone panel evaluation includes lipid profile, thyroid assessment, analysis of your sex steroids including total estrogen, progesterone, free testosterone, pregnenolone, and DHEA sulfate, and adrenal testing.

Neurotransmitters

These are crucial for proper brain function. Low levels of neurotransmitters cause increased pain and fatigue. They are growth regulators. Thyroid hormones help in brain development. To detect thyroid disorders, I would suggest testing for decreased brain neurotransmitters. Immunohistochemical mapping of brain triiodothyronine shows hormone concentrations clearly. Combined biochemical and morphologic data helps you detect thyroid hormone activity levels. High concentrations of locus coeruleus nor-epinephrine promote active conversion of thyroxin (T4) to triiodothyronine (T3).

Glutathione

Glutathione is very effective for autoimmune diseases. These are available as supplements. It is difficult to absorb orally. It can regenerate other antioxidants like vitamins C and E. It is a very useful nutrient for intestinal health and is essential for glutathione formation. It contains lots of anti-oxidants and hence is very useful in treating chronic thyroid conditions.

Inflammation

An inflammation test is important for people with thyroid disorders as chronic thyroid conditions cause inflammation. Blood tests to detect inflammation include C-reactive protein, erythrocyte sedimentation rate, and plasma viscosity. Inflammation in any part of your body causes release of extra protein from inflamed part. This circulates in the blood. These blood tests can detect such increases and thereby detect inflammation. However, these are elementary tests. High levels indicate need to dwell deeper into causes and detect actual problem.

===\\\===\\\===\\\===\\\===\\\===\\\===

60. Cold Laser Therapy or Low-level Laser Therapy

Cold Laser Therapy or Low Level Laser Therapy (LLLT) is a treatment option that utilizes light in specific wavelengths to interact with body tissue. This treatment is very effective at relieving pain and swelling. It improves functionality of body organs and reduces spasms. Cold laser therapy should not be used on pregnant women and on cancerous lesions.

Working of Cold Lasers

Cold lasers are handheld devices around the size of a flashlight. Both you and your doctor should use protective glasses during therapy treatment sessions. Each session lasts for ten minutes. The beam is applied by a therapist, doctor, or qualified technician.

Normally, laser is placed directly over affected area for a minimum of thirty seconds. Depending on dosage of laser unit and area under treatment, time is adjusted. When laser is held over affected region, non-thermal photons of light emitted from laser pass through your skin and penetrate deep within. This light can penetrate two to five centimeters below the skin.

When laser beam is passed over body tissue, enzymes within the cell absorb light energy. Mitochondria absorbs visible red light and infrared light is absorbed at cell membrane. This increases ATP levels and DNA production increases. Membrane stability improves. Flow of ions improves and cell metabolism stabilizes. Once absorbed, this light energy sets off a chain of functions like reducing pain or/and inflammation, increasing intracellular metabolism, and repairing injured or damaged tissue. Overall healing speeds up.

The laser light irradiation increases production of collagen and epithelial tissue. New capillaries are produced and their density increases. Nerve regeneration is stimulated. Muscles relax. There is remarked reduction in pain and inflammation. Laser therapy also improves functioning of immune system and responses improve.

Advantages of Cold Laser Therapy

□ Cold Laser Therapy is a non-invasive procedure as there is no need for any surgical invasion.

□ It is antiviral and antifungal.

□ It improves drainage in lymph. This improves blood circulation and promotes overall healing.

□ Cold Laser Therapy process does not require any medications and hence you do not suffer from any side effects of medications.

□ It induces production of natural painkillers or endorphins in your body and thereby reduces pain.

□ There is no specific recovery time as it is not a surgery.

□ Cold Laser Therapy relaxes tight muscles and you find relief from chronic pain. These tight muscles restrict mobility and are responsible for pain in joints.

□ The therapy does not cause any side effects.

▫ Cold Laser Therapy promotes release of anti-inflammatory enzymes and suppresses inflammatory enzymes that cause pain, swelling, and redness.

▫ Cold Laser Therapy stimulates fibroblastic and osteoblastic proliferation. This helps repair bone tissue.

Disadvantages of Cold Laser Therapy

▫ Cold Laser Therapy requires numerous sittings, sometimes even as many as thirty.

▫ It does not provide immediate relief from pain. You have to take up as many as ten sittings to find little relief from pain or inflammation.

▫ You should schedule sittings of two to four each week.

▫ Sometimes, old injuries are aggravated.

▫ Major insurance companies do not offer coverage for this treatment.

Cold Laser Therapy for Hypothyroidism

If you are hypothyroid, your thyroid gland is not functioning properly; rather, it is not producing sufficient amount of thyroid hormones. Cold laser therapy if properly administered and carried out can improve your hypothyroid symptoms substantially. You should ideally undergo a treatment session of ten weeks. You can thereafter stay away from thyroid supplements. Further, it also improves your immune system. This acts positively on your thyroid disorder.

Reviewing Cold Laser Therapy

This is a new therapy and adopts new techniques to tackle various ailments. This therapy is slowly gaining acceptance as a complementary form of medical treatment. You can use this therapy in isolation or in combination with other treatment options. It is a good alternative to invasive treatment. It is considered a reasonable and acceptable treatment option for certain types of pain by most health care professionals.

However, it need not be used as an alternative to conventional treatments like magnetic therapy, ultrasound, interferential therapy, and others. It can be effectively used in treatment of thyroid disorders. It delivers results due to reaction between laser and irradiated biological tissue.

It is an extremely safe treatment option. Laser light radiation does not affect healthy cells. It rather restores energy and nutrient levels, balances body functions, and improves oxygen permeability to sick cells. This speeds up regeneration and healing of tissues. However, this therapy treatment should be explored further to dwell deeper into greater possibilities of widening options for better treatment.

However, extensive research is required to determine ideal durations of treatment, most suitable wavelengths, dose, and perfect location of treatment. Range also needs to be ascertained to arrive at specific limit such that pain and inflammation in nerves and joints are well addressed.

===\\\===\\\===\\\===\\\===\\\===\\\===

61. Exercises for Minimizing Symptoms of Your Thyroid Disorders

Exercises are good for every individual, more so if you have any thyroid disorders like hypothyroidism, hyperthyroidism, and others. Often hypothyroid people are unable to diagnose their illness in the early stages. Hence, they put on lot of weight. Normally hyperthyroid people lose weight due to high metabolism. Nonetheless, with regular medication, you often become hypothyroid and start putting on weight. Irrespective of everything, it is essential to include exercises within your daily routine.

Benefits of Exercises for Thyroid Patients

Thyroid gland produces two important hormones- triiodothyronine and thyroxin. These hormones are responsible for extensive cell activities like protein synthesis, metabolic rate regulation, vitamin metabolism, and many others. Exercises can improve circulation of these hormones throughout your body.

If you are hyperthyroid, weight bearing exercises are extremely beneficial. These improve muscle tone and help maintain bone density. If you are hypothyroid, exercises stimulate metabolic rate and reduce weight gain. Regular exercises also improve functioning of immune system, reduce stress levels, and improve your energy levels.

Exercises for Hypothyroidism

Hypothyroidism causes excessive weight gain, in some cases uncontrollable weight gain. Hence, you should adopt an exercise plan that suits your condition in consultation with your doctor. It is best to adopt an intensive exercise plan to reduce body weight. Jogging, walking, swimming, and aerobic exercises are good choices. Whatever you choose, stick to a routine, and follow it diligently. Only then, you can find results.

Exercises for Hyperthyroidism

Hyperthyroid people should adopt moderate or low-intensity exercises. It is best to stay away from high-intensity exercises, as your body will react negatively to such exercises. Suitable exercises include:

Weight Bearing Exercises
Push-ups are ideal exercises for your condition. Start slowly by doing push-ups while keeping both hands and knees on the floor. Repeat in sets of ten, thrice each day.

Aerobics
Step aerobics is best suited for your condition. Choose a step and set it to the lowest level. Practice this step at specified level until you are comfortable. Thereafter, increase the level and do it accordingly. This is a very effective cardiovascular workout. Practice aerobic exercises for twenty minutes each day.

Yoga
Yoga is a stress buster. It not only relaxes but also energizes your body. Simple yoga poses include fish pose to provide essential nutrients to head, chest, thyroid gland and neck, cat pose to improve blood circulation to spine, and bridge pose to relax entire body and improve brain functions.

Other low-intensity exercises for hyperthyroidism include brisk walking, swimming, and cycling.

Avoid exercising for long durations at a stretch. Break down your exercise routine into simple and smaller segments spread across the day. However, exercises alone cannot bring in expected benefits. In order to overcome thyroid disorders, you should also adopt specific lifestyle changes.

===\\\===\\\===\\\===\\\===\\\===\\\===

62. Thyroid Care - The Role of Chiropractors in Managing Thyroid Disease

Hypothyroidism causes various musculoskeletal problems like poor recovery from muscle injury, carpal tunnel syndrome, and autoimmune joint diseases of arthritis or joint degeneration, back pain due to obesity, inflammation, and headaches. Visit a chiropractor to seek remedial measures to overcome these.

Who is a Chiropractor?

Chiropractors are trained health professionals. A chiropractic doctor is trained in varied techniques including spinal manipulation and differential diagnosis. Differential diagnosis is the process of evaluating a medical problem in terms of its underlying causes and related health issues.

Chiropractors use various non-surgical treatment options like spinal manipulation and mobilization. They do not use drugs, surgery, or other medications. Instead, they dwell on dietary and nutritional aspects of any ailment and suggest suitable options by correcting irregularities in these.

Chiropractors are registered primary healthcare providers in every major state in the United States. They have professional and legal responsibilities to properly diagnose their patients and suggest suitable treatment. They analyze your medical history, conduct a thorough physical examination, and go through various laboratory and imaging test reports to eventually diagnose your ailment and suggest suitable corrective measures.

Thyroid Disorders and Chiropractor

Most thyroid disorders occur due to poor lifestyle habits, dietary imbalances, and insufficient nutritional intake. People with autoimmune ailments and Hashimoto's thyroiditis suffer from vitamin D imbalances, blood sugar, gluten sensitivity, intestinal permeability, and similar others. Musculoskeletal pain is a major symptom of hypothyroidism and chiropractors can resolve your problem through appropriate massages and proper spinal care.

Hyperthyroid people or those with Graves' disease are at a serious risk of suffering a stroke due to overactive thyroid conditions. They often suffer from related problems like migraines, vertigo, muscular spasms, and similar others. These are not ailments or diseases in the strictest sense; rather they can be easily addressed through significant changes in dietary habits, nutritional status, and lifestyle patterns. Chiropractors are well qualified and equipped to advise you on these issues effectively.

Thyroid Care is an Inherent Part of Chiropractic Care

Thyroid gland is the major organ that controls almost all important body functions. Thyroid hormones maintain body temperature, rate of energy production; regulate growth hormones, mental development, and overall health. Low thyroid production affects every aspect of your body. Thyroid disorders often remain undiagnosed in early stages as most symptoms overlap with other ailments. Sometimes treatments for other ailments provide relief albeit only for a short period and symptoms surface again with greater veracity. This also causes chronic inflammation and immune deregulation. An in-depth clinical examination thereupon hints at thyroid disorders. By this time, your thyroid problem is more acute and you require proper treatment.

A chiropractor is your best bet here, as chiropractors do not prescribe any medications or hormone supplements. They provide suitable remedies by attacking the root cause of your thyroid disorder. They determine the chemical or mechanical factors responsible for your ailments and address these. Changes in your diet and lifestyle can restore such chemical imbalances.

Chiropractic treatment does not address a single issue; rather it treats your entire body system as a whole and does not suggest medical solutions for specific ailment alone. Thyroid disorders affect every body system; some acutely while some others marginally. Consequently normal body functioning is disturbed and your physiological, biomechanical, and biochemical functions suffer. Nervous system is affected. Your quality of life worsens. Sometimes you develop newer diseases. Your mental health suffers and you feel depressed.

Why Go to a Chiropractor?

Chiropractors are clinically educated and trained to handle problems developing due to thyroid malfunctions. They can accurately identify actual causes for your physiological disturbances. They use nutritional compounds, dietary changes, and devise appropriate lifestyle management to guide your deregulated physiology back within the correct and healthy ranges of good health. Your body responds positively to conventional chiropractic remedies and care. You are in safe hands once you approach a chiropractor for your thyroid problems.

Medical practitioners focus more on thyroid replacement options like medications, surgical measures, and similar others. They harp on thyroid-stimulating hormone (TSH) as the main factor to be considered to restore normal thyroid health. However, this alone is not the remedy to your problem. Lifestyle, diet, and nutrition are extremely important factors for patients suffering from thyroid conditions. Most often, these remain unaddressed and ignored.

Often, taming an autoimmune thyroid condition through dietary and lifestyle adjustments is a better solution to handle your ailment. Many elderly people are unable to bear the severe side effects of medications or withstand the psychological effects of surgery. Chiropractic solutions can repeatedly put most thyroid symptoms into a state of remission. These can greatly improve quality of life through better functioning of most body organs. Further, they also prevent autoimmune diseases from developing in future.

Visiting a chiropractor not only cures your thyroid problems, it assures you of better health and well-being.

===\\\===\\\===\\\===\\\===\\\===\\\===

Part-VII: Preventing and Coping with Thyroid Disorders

63. Five Steps to Preventing Thyroid Disease

Irrespective of whether you have thyroid disease, inculcate the following to stay protected and improve thyroid function:

1. Iodine Consumption: Monitor your consumption of iodine. Too little and too much of iodine affect your thyroid gland negatively. The recommended daily intake for a healthy adult is 120 to 150 mcg. It is much less for babies and children and higher for pregnant and lactating women. Normally, you get necessary iodine from iodized salt. Sea salt is also available in iodized forms. Use such salt. Intermittently consume seafood like seaweed. Eating tuna is good but do not eat it daily as it increases mercury levels. This leads to thyroid problems. Consuming too much of kelp or bladder wrack increases chances of hypothyroidism or goiter. If you live in areas that lack iodine, take an iodine multi containing around 100 mcg of iodine.

2. Soy: Soy Contains Isoflavones. This causes thyroid problems. Excessive soy isoflavones worsen hypothyroidism, thyroid nodules, and goiter. Restrict consumption of soy products and supplements like powders, smoothies, creams, or pills. Eat soy food in moderation, just a small single serving daily. Further, it is better to eat soy in its natural form as present in tofu, miso soup, or tempeh. Overconsumption of soy transforms it into a drug. It strains your immune system and it could trigger thyroid problems. Do not feed any soy-based formulas to infants as this could lead to thyroid diseases later in life.

3. Smoking: Stop smoking if you are a smoker and do not start if you do not smoke. Cigarette smoke contains various toxins like thiocyanate. This not only triggers thyroid disease in susceptible people but also damages your thyroid. Smokers are at a greater risk of developing eye complications like those present in people with Graves' disease. Further, any medical treatment is less effective in smokers as toxins present in cigarettes inhibit medications. These toxins worsen existing thyroid problems.

4. Fluoride: Fluoride is used as a drug to treat hyperthyroidism as it reduces over activity of thyroid gland. If you have a normal thyroid, be careful of using excessive fluoridated treatments or products containing fluoride. Most dental products like rinses, washes, and toothpastes contain fluoride. If you are a hypothyroid, do not use toothpastes with fluoride. Stay away from tap water, instead, use and drink bottled water as tap water contains fluoride. Fluoride as present in tap water and toothpastes can further reduce thyroid gland activity. This will lower your already low levels of thyroid hormones.

5. Maintain Balanced Ph Levels in Body: A healthy thyroid assures overall good health. If your thyroid does not function normally, metabolism is irregular. Acid accumulates in body due to poor digestion and cellular activity. Body cells are full of acid that needs to be excreted. If you consume more acid-forming substances, the problem deteriorates further. Thyroid problems affect functioning of your immune system. Body immunity levels drop and you develop infections. Some infections turn chronic. Acid accumulation coupled with poor immunity levels further reduces your body's ability to neutralize acids. When acid waste accumulates in your bloodstream, essential substances like oxygen and glucose are unable to move in your blood. Thyroid gland function is hampered. To restore thyroid gland function and remove acidic waste from your body, include more alkaline foods and minerals in your diet.

Regular exercises, maintaining a steady lifestyle, overcoming stress, educating yourself on thyroid disorders and possible problems, and adopting remedial measures help you prevent and combat thyroid better.

===\\\===\\\===\\\===\\\===\\\===\\\===

64. Ten Easy Ways to Avoid or Delay the Onset of Thyroid Disease

Thyroid disorders are very common. Often misdiagnosed and misunderstood, it is possible to delay or avoid thyroid diseases. As with virtually every bodily function, your diet holds the key to good thyroid health. There are specific foods that you should eat and specific foods, which you should avoid.

Simple ways to manage and maintain good thyroid health include:

1. Include lots of fresh fruits of different colors and vegetables like green spinach, broccoli, and leafy vegetables in your daily diet. These are high in antioxidants and help maintain good health. Antioxidants help your body neutralize oxidative stress that could otherwise damage your thyroid. Kelp, a dense sea vegetable, purifies your blood and contains natural iodine. It is helpful in treating thyroid disorders.

2. Trace amounts of minerals like copper, iron, and zinc are important for healthy thyroid functions. Iron and copper deficiency hampers thyroid hormone production. Low levels of zinc lowers TSH levels. Leafy green vegetables, shellfish, beans, red meat, and poultry are high in iron. Oysters, organ meats, cashews, clams, sunflower seeds, crabs, whole-grain products, wheat bran cereals, and cocoa products are rich in copper. Consume foods like mushrooms, calf's liver, turnip greens, and Swiss chard. These provide essential quantities of such minerals. Include more of vitamin C foods like red berries, citrus fruits, tomatoes, bell peppers, and potatoes to maximize iron absorption efficiency of your body.

3. Selenium is important not only to produce T3 hormone but also to regulate it within your body. Selenium helps in normal functioning of thyroid gland. Good sources of selenium include tuna, shrimp, Brazil nuts, cod, calf's liver, and halibut. Turkey, a lean protein, is low in calories. It also contains selenium. It improves functioning of immune system and metabolism of thyroid hormone.

4. Soy, high in isoflavones, is a goitrogen food. Soymilk, soybean oil, soy burgers, and processed soy foods lead to decreased thyroid function. Restricting or avoiding soy foods is good for your thyroid. Nonetheless, you can eat fermented soy foods like tempeh, brewed soy sauce, and miso as fermentation reduces goitrogenic content of isoflavones.

5. Coconut oil and butter contain raw unsaturated fatty acids that help manage weight gain and increase metabolism rate. Your body is able to metabolize these fats quickly and efficiently. This helps and regulates thyroid functions smoothly.

6. Stay away from goitrogen foods as these suppress functioning of thyroid gland. They also enlarge your thyroid gland leading to goiter. Such foods include peanuts and peanut butter, broccoli, cabbage, cauliflower, Brussels sprouts, kale, mustard, turnips, and canola oil.

7. If you have food allergies like those of wheat products, milk products including cheese, milk, and ice cream, you are susceptible to thyroid disorders. Your thyroid often remains undiagnosed as symptoms of food allergies and thyroid disorders are similar and common.

8. Avoid canned or processed foods as these suppress digestive enzymes in your body. Avoid refined grains like white flour as bran and germ of such grains has been removed and hence their fiber and

mineral content is very low. Also, you should avoid white bread and bleached pastas.

9. Side effects of many medications lead to thyroid problems. Monitor your medications, read warning labels on medications, and consult your doctor to understand possible complications. Avoid exposure to radiation through x-rays or radiation treatment for other ailments like cancer.

10. Avoid smoking and consuming alcohol. These not only affect thyroid health but also your general health.

===\\\===\\\===\\\===\\\===\\\===\\\===

65. Caring for a Person Having a Thyroid Disease

Thyroid disorders are very common. Women are more prone to thyroid problems than men are. Thyroid is not only about weight gain or loss. Thyroid disorders can be broadly classified as hypothyroidism, hyperthyroidism, and cancer of the thyroid gland.

Thyroid gland is the master of all glands in your body. It controls important processes like metabolism, growth, and various functions of nervous system. You should have proper balance of thyroid hormone. Only then, you feel well and can live well. Any change in thyroid hormone secretion affects your well-being extensively. Excess thyroid hormone secretion or hyperthyroidism increases your heartbeat rate immensely. You feel anxious and nervous. You feel hungry always. Although you eat a lot, you seem to be losing weight extensively. You are unable to sleep peacefully and you feel irritated always. Poor sleep combined with high-energy levels exhaust you both physically and mentally.

If your thyroid hormone level is low, you feel tired eternally. Any small work seems to be a huge task and you feel exhausted and worn-out. You feel bad and depressed about your condition. You try your best to overcome your weakness; however, this makes you feel all the more tired and exhausted. You keep putting on weight despite being very strict about your food habits and exercises.

If you have thyroid cancer, it increases your anxiety even more. Although doctors declare thyroid cancer as very mild, yet, being cancer-affected provokes a frightening feeling. Often surgery is the best option for thyroid cancer. However, undergoing surgery is not a simple task. It takes a huge toll on your mental strength.

Even though thyroid is considered to be a mild and easily treatable disease, those affected by thyroid suffer various problems. Hence, if your friend or family member has thyroid disorders, understand what they are going through, as it is not possible to put down their agony in words. It is a challenging disease and you should remain compassionate and patient while interacting with such affected people. Help them relax and enjoy life in their own way.

===\\\===\\\===\\\===\\\===\\\===\\\===

66. What Type of Care is the Best for a Thyroid Disease Patient?

Thyroid disorders disrupt your life to a great extent. Nonetheless, you should be able to devise suitable ways of overcoming this disruption and live your life normally.

The Best Care for a Thyroid Disease Patient

Keep in mind simple facts like:

1. Thyroid is extremely stressful. The best way to handle this stress is to stay healthy. Eat nutritious food, exercise, go for walks, and give sufficient rest to body. Sleep well. Follow a set pattern of life and adhere to it religiously.

2. Practice yoga and meditation. Push away depressing and doubtful thoughts from your mind. Focus your energy on meditation. Adopt healing techniques like guided imagery and hypnosis to control and maintain a proper mind and body synchronization.

Yoga improves your concentration. It helps you tackle problems arising due to high or low energy levels.

3. Seek help of a qualified and experienced psychotherapist to address your problems of anxiety and depression. Psychotherapist with a strong background in mind-body approaches can provide remedial measures to handle such problems.

4. Seek help from support groups. Often people with thyroid problems come together to form support groups. Since members of such groups experience similar problems, you can share your experiences and feelings. Such communication proves very helpful in overcoming stress and depression.

5. Your family and friends prove to be a pillar of support in fighting off thyroid problems. Discuss your problems and limitations frankly with family members. Draft out plans to overcome these limitations.

Keep your family informed and educated about thyroid disorders. Spend quiet time with your spouse and loved ones to keep your mind and body happy and content.

6. Stay aware of your TSH levels. Check regularly to see if these numbers are constant or fluctuating. Visit your doctor regularly and give updates on recent developments. This helps doctor analyze your situation and advise accordingly. Continue medications as prescribed by your doctor.

7. Radiation should be avoided. If going for a mammography or dental x-rays, use a protective cover for your neck. Radiation and x-rays affect your thyroid gland negatively.

8. Take thyroid medication at the same time each day. If you follow a pattern of having your thyroid medicines first thing in the morning or after breakfast and your TSH levels are normal, adhere to it diligently. Be disciplined in your approach to tackle your thyroid better.

9. Stay positive. Depression, anxiety, and panic are common in people with thyroid. Often, you feel demoralized for not being able to recollect properly. Sometimes, you are unable to perform to your capacity. This upsets your morale. It is important to set aside

depressing thoughts and focus on what you are able to do. This not only improves your focus but also boosts your self-confidence and self-esteem.

===\\\===\\\===\\\===\\\===\\\===\\\===

67. Ten Practical Tips for Thyroid Disease Caregivers

A caregiver is one who looks after a sick person. Thyroid disorders lead to depression, anxiety, hyper-energetic, mood swings, and various medical complications. As a caregiver, you should help the person overcome physical and mental limitations occurring due to thyroid disorders.

Some practical tips for thyroid disease caregivers include:

1. If you are a caregiver to your family member or friend, analyze medical condition in your own way. It is important to give full attention to what doctors and specialists have diagnosed and prescribed. At the same time, also listen to your gut feeling and instincts, as you can understand your family member's symptoms and problems on a personal basis.

2. Dwell deep into the actual cause of thyroid problem. Remain aware of what could be the consequences of thyroid disorder as it progresses or how best to handle its limitations. This keeps you prepared for any emergencies.

3. Analyze and understand the extent to which your family member is dependent or independent. Strategize your care giving accordingly. Care giving does not mean doing everything for your loved one. Allow sufficient space and time for your loved one to do things themselves. This boosts their self-confidence, a prime factor to recover from thyroid disorders. Take help of technology and other strategies to offer as much independence as possible.

4. If you are a caregiver working outside your home, you need to plan and juggle office and home responsibilities. This is not easy. Delegate the work and responsibilities among family members and friends. Do not feel shy to ask or accept help.

5. Being a caregiver does not mean you forget to take care of yourself. Eat balanced meals regularly. Sleep for a minimum of eight hours at night. This keeps you energized to take care of your family member or friend.

6. Understand your limitations. You should plan caring schedules accordingly. If you have to attend to any important, work or go somewhere, seek help of neighbors, extended family, or friends to look after the ailing member. Remain realistic of how much time you can devote to your family member. Discuss with doctors and other family members on the best way to manage the situation.

7. Relaxation is of paramount importance to you as a caregiver. Unless you are relaxed and calm, you cannot provide as much care and love to your family member with thyroid. Set aside at least thirty minutes each day to do things you like and enjoy, be it gardening, reading, knitting, or any other hobby. Take an extended break over the weekend or once in a fortnight. Ask your friend or neighbor to fill in while you are away.

8. Join a support group of caregivers of thyroid patients. Meet members of such support groups regularly. Thyroid symptoms are varied and different. Discuss and get to know how others take care of thyroid patients in similar situations.

9. Visit your doctor regularly. You should schedule appointments for your regular checkups. Unless you are healthy, you cannot be a good caregiver. Discuss your concerns and responsibilities as a caregiver with your doctor. Get recommended immunizations and screenings.

10. Care giving is rewarding and yet stressful. Physical workload increases and mental exhaustion is also extensive. It could also cause financial constraints. Seek help from friends and other family members to handle financial exigencies. Be clear of what the present requirements are and what could develop in future.

===\\\===\\\===\\\===\\\===\\\===\\\===

Part-VIII: Lifestyle Changes and Self-Help for Thyroid Disease

68. Ten Lifestyle Changes for Better Thyroid Health

Thyroid is a very small gland. It is important to maintain a healthy thyroid to stay healthy. Lifestyle changes for better thyroid health include:

1. Eat a balanced diet rich in proteins, magnesium, calcium, selenium, and iodine. These help your thyroid function normally. Brazil nuts and walnuts contain high amounts of selenium. Restrict intake of goitrogen foods. These hamper thyroid hormone production. Such foods include cruciferous vegetables like cabbage, cauliflower, and Brussels sprouts, soy, and peanuts. Limit soy products. Salt, beets, garlic, and turnips supply iodine.

2. Stress disrupts thyroid functioning. Stress releases cortisol. Chronic stress causes high levels of cortisol in blood. Reduce stress. Adopt relaxing techniques like meditation, hot water baths, tai chi, massage, nature walks, and acupuncture to lower stress levels and enable thyroid to stay healthy.

3. Maintain adequate iron levels in body. Iron helps thyroid hormones T3 and T4 to function normally. Low iron levels often cause hypothyroidism. Consume iron-rich foods regularly.

4. Refrain from foods made of refined flour. This flour is processed and it contains bromine. This mineral hampers thyroid production. Eat flour of whole grains and cereals.

5. Thyroid causes inflammation and lowers immunity levels. Increase intake of cold-water fish like tuna, salmon, halibut, herring, lake

trout, flounder, and sardines. These are rich sources of omega-3 fatty acids. These acids help brain functions and increase immunity levels.

6. Include tomatoes, sea vegetables, seaweed, squash, and bell peppers in your daily diet. These vegetables have high fiber and are low in calories. They help manage your weight and thyroid problems. Eat fiber-rich fruits like cherries, berries, citrus fruits, cantaloupe, kiwi, papaya, plums, mango, and red grapes. Choose fruits over juices to maintain blood sugar levels.

7. Take your thyroid medicines on an empty stomach with a glass of water. Do not eat or drink anything for half an hour. Avoid iron and calcium supplements and high-fiber foods for four hours as they impair your body's ability to absorb thyroid medicines.

8. Yoga is very beneficial for maintain normal thyroid health. Specific yoga poses like bridge pose, king pigeon pose, plow pose, shoulder stand, full boat pose, and upward-facing two-foot staff pose increase flow of blood to thyroid. Seek help from a yoga expert to practice these poses correctly.

9. Exercise regularly. Exercise stimulates thyroid hormone and increases metabolic rate. This is helpful for hypothyroids. If you are a hyperthyroid, exercise soothes your nerves and lowers stress levels. Follow a regular routine of exercise. Swimming, walking, jogging, and running are all good forms of exercise.

10. Include herbs like kelp, guggul, Irish moss, and ashwagandha to balance hormonal deficiency and support adrenal function. Guggul relieves joint pain and osteoarthritis. These herbs reduce cholesterol and triglycerides levels and help reduce weight.

===\\\===\\\===\\\===\\\===\\\===\\\===

69. Staying Positive and Informed

Thyroid imbalance is not a difficult condition to treat; however, the symptoms and treatments transform it into a difficult condition for you. Nonetheless, gathering information about your ailment and reacting with a positive attitude goes a long way in handling thyroid imbalance effectively.

Tips to Remain Positive

Some simple tips for being positive and informed are:

◻ Staying positive in a medical situation is difficult; yet it is important to realize that being positive increases your body vibrations and helps you tackle debilitating situations better.

◻ Garner your thoughts and focus only on situations you want to happen in your life.

◻ Meditate regularly as meditation increases and improves your focus. Your mental energies surge and you remain positive.

◻ Visualize about happy tidings and experiences in your life. This keeps your mood in a positive upbeat and lets you experience positive events.

◻ Think about the present and do not keep thinking of the future or the past. Remaining in the present will help you to relax and feel free.

◻ Listen to music of your liking. This soothes your mind and improves your mood.

◻ Love yourself and appreciate your efforts. This improves your state of mind.

Stay Informed

◻ Thyroid imbalances even if rectified can pop up any time in your life. Hence, it is best to choose a medical practitioner with whom you are comfortable and feel at ease to discuss all your problems. The best way to do this is to look up recommendations of similar thyroid patients at websites. Read these and choose accordingly.

◻ Scout the Internet and learn all about your thyroid imbalance. Thyroid disorder is not a straightforward disease; it presents differently across different people. Analyze your symptoms and laboratory reports. Gather information based on similar situations. Remaining informed about your position makes it simpler to handle symptoms. It also prepares you to handle emergencies better.

◻ Form a support system or become a member of an existing one. This is easier said than done. Thyroid diseases pose varied symptoms and most symptoms are common to many ailments like depression, sleeping problems, anxiety, mood swings, hair loss, irritability, weight problems, and many others. Hence, seeking people with similar medical situations like yours could be difficult. Yet, try to discuss with such people. Visit online thyroid disease bulletin boards, chat rooms, and forums. This provides a deeper insight into actual situations and helps you stay informed of what could happen. You meet and discuss with people who have passed through almost same situations.

□ Analyze your situation and concentrate on the most important and difficult symptoms. This not only increases your focus but also channelizes your energy to handle your symptoms and thyroid conditions better. Choose the best option to tackle your disease in the most effective manner.

===\\\===\\\===\\\===\\\===\\\===\\\===

70. Taking Care of Yourself - Healthy Living with Thyroid Disease

Living with thyroid condition does not mean you cannot lead a normal life. You can lead a healthy and happy life if you adhere to simple caring tips:

1. Gather as much information as possible about your thyroid condition. Remain aware of possible limitations and medical emergencies. Read books, scout the Internet, and discuss your condition with doctors to understand your position.

2. Be regular with your medications. Take medicines at the same time each day as this proves to be more effective. It takes some time for thyroid hormone replacement pills to take effect. Be patient and adhere to pill dosage and timing. Go for regular checkups and follow-ups.

3. Eat healthy food. Sit down and enjoy your meals. Do not eat on the run as then you do not chew and eat well. Half-eaten or unchewed food only adds to your weight and does not provide essential nutrition. Eat balanced meals regularly. Never skip meals. Eat in moderation. Do not eat large portions. Be sure that fruits, vegetables, lean proteins, whole grain foods, and low-fat dairy products constitute major portion of each meal.

4. You should exercise regularly. Your thyroid condition, be it hypothyroid or hyperthyroid, improves with exercise. Weight changes can be easily controlled with exercise. Choose any exercise form you like and feel comfortable. Swimming, jogging, walking, aerobic exercises, yoga, and simple physical workouts are all good forms of

exercise. You may exercise at home or go to a gym. Prioritize exercise as a regular habit and follow a schedule diligently.

5. Stress is an inherent part of your existence. Learn to manage stress such that it does not control your life. Stress affects your performance levels. Further, thyroid imbalances create stressful situations due to mood swings and hyper energy levels. Excessive stress often leads to depression and hypertension. Adopt relaxation techniques like yoga, reading a book, listening to music, gardening, playing with pets, and similar others.

6. A good night's sleep is of paramount importance. Lack of sleep can jeopardize your thyroid condition further. Without sufficient sleep, you feel tired, grumpy, depressed, and lethargic. Despite pressing work schedules, follow regular sleep patterns and adhere to it religiously. Sleep and wake at almost the same time each day, even on off-days and weekends. Avoid stimulating work just before going to sleep. Similarly, refrain from watching television before going to bed.

7. Analyze your health regularly. It is true that a small pill taken once each day handles your thyroid imbalance. Yet, it is good to do a self-evaluation of how you feel. Sit and think if you feel depressed, fatigued, or energized. Analyze existing symptoms and check if there is any improvement. Further, understand your body and gauge its requirements, as you are the best person to judge yourself.

8. Remain alert of your medical condition. Seek help from your family members, friends, and neighbors. Also, seek help from support groups. These people are experiencing similar medical condition as yours and can understand your problems well. If you are feeling jittery or anxious, pour out your worries and seek their help. Do not bolt up all emotions within you as this causes immense strain on your nervous system. This also upsets your thyroid condition.

Thyroid could prove a difficult condition to be in; yet tackling it healthily can help you overcome thyroid imbalances effectively, efficiently, and easily.

===\\\===\\\===\\\===\\\===\\\===\\\===

A Final Note - Why Should You Call Dr. Jeff Smith's Office to Get the Help on Thyroid Immediately?

Do you suffer from any of these symptoms?

- Frequent indigestion
- Chronic pain
- Feel bloated after eating
- Constipation
- Fatigue
- Frequent loose bowel movements
- Repetitive vomiting
- Mouth ulcers or sores

These symptoms are due to malfunctioning of your thyroid gland. Your thyroid is a small, butterfly-shaped gland located in your lower neck. This minuscule gland secretes two hormones, T3 and T4. These two hormones are not only responsible for all metabolic functions of your body but also support your physical and mental growth. Excess or deficient secretion of these hormones may cause a multitude of ailments and associated problems.

Often, thyroid diseases are not diagnosed at all, rather they are misdiagnosed and you undergo treatment for ailments you do not suffer from. Are you tired of trying different drugs and medications, which do not provide any relief at all? Do not ignore these symptoms. You should visit Dr. Jeff Smith's clinic immediately. We determine the root cause for your discomfort and repetitive occurrence of such symptoms. Regular health checkups are important.

Why go to Dr. Jeff Smith's clinic only?

If you suspect you have a thyroid disease, it is best to have a complete medical check-up. Dr. Jeff Smith's clinic is one of the few clinics in Bentonville, Arkansas that attacks the source of your problem. We use a combined functional, metabolic, and neurological protocol to determine actual cause of peripheral neuropathy. This functional approach provides you permanent relief from the regular thyroid symptoms of fatigue and pain.

What are Thyroid Diseases?

Thyroid diseases affect more than twenty seven million Americans. However, thyroid diseases are often either not diagnosed properly or just ignored. It is a fact that more than half of affected American population does not even know of their ailment. Women are more susceptible to thyroid disorders. Almost one in every five women will suffer from thyroid problems at some point in their lives. Some may not even be aware of their ailment.

Hypothyroidism or underactive thyroid is the most common thyroid disease. Your thyroid gland produces insufficient amount of thyroid hormone. Symptoms are mild and few at first. However, left untreated hypothyroidism manifests into a major ailment and is responsible for joint pain, obesity, goiter, and heart ailments. Although iodine deficiency is the primary cause for hypothyroidism, sometimes an autoimmune disease, Hashimoto's thyroiditis, also causes hypothyroidism. Early diagnosis and treatment is important.
If your thyroid gland produces excess hormones, it is hyperthyroidism.

Visit Dr. Jeff Smith for a No Obligation Initial Consultation

If you want to improve your health through chiropractic and holistic therapies, our clinic is the correct place to be. We have been using holistic techniques and medicines for more than fifteen years to help people maintain good health. Our team at The Thyroid Relief

Bentonville Clinic is always present to analyze your symptoms, conduct a full thyroid hormone panel, and provide suitable treatment. It is very simple to arrange a no obligation initial consultation with Dr. Smith. Just read on...

Fix the Appointment Today

It will take just five minutes or even less to plan an appointment with Dr. Smith. You only need to call, send an email, or drop by our clinic. Our team will fix an appointment that fits within your schedule comfortably. You are almost on the path to good health!

What's in no obligation initial consultation with Dr. Smith?

Dr. Smith will meet you personally at your appointment in no obligation initial consultation and inquire about your symptoms. Thereafter Dr. Smith will explain how chiropractic therapy and medication can absolve your problems. You can question him on any doubts regarding chiropractic therapy. Be rest assured, all your doubts and queries will be answered patiently. The holistic approach to treating a disorder is in its nascent stage. Many people are unaware of how simple things we often overlook in our fast-paced lives can affect our health drastically. Mr. Smith lays bare such facts for you to understand and assimilate.

What is the cost of such treatment?

Every case is individualistic and cost of treatment differs across cases. Dr. Smith will chart out your treatment outline and schedule according to your medical health. It is easy to alter your lifestyle habits and work out simple ways to overcome hormonal imbalances. Medication is not always necessary; Dr. Smith suggests easily available foods to improve and encourage better thyroid health.

What are you waiting for?

Get started right now. Visit our website and fill in the contact form. You can also call us and our representative will schedule an appointment that suits you the best. Your health is of prime importance, just book the call. You will be happy that you fixed the appointment with Dr. Smith and entrusted your health to him!

===\\\===\\\===\\\===\\\===\\\===\\\===

www.ingramcontent.com/pod-product-compliance
Lightning Source LLC
Chambersburg PA
CBHW071416170526
45165CB00001B/301